HEADACHES THAT
PERSIST

*14+ years of research on headaches,
migraines & rare headaches*

*Reviewed by headache neurologists devoted exclusively to
managing headache pain.*

Brent Lucas, B.A.
Headache Researcher

T0062370

Help for Headaches
London, Canada
2009
www.headache-help.org

Graphic design by:
Chameleon Creative: www.chameleoncreative.com
MLS Graphic Design: www.mlsgraphicdesign.ca

Our mission is to efficiently provide the world's finest, most comprehensive book publishing service, enabling every author to experience success. To find out how to publish your book, your way, and have it available worldwide, visit us online at www.trafford.com

Trafford rev. 9/17/2009

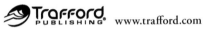 www.trafford.com

North America & international
toll-free: 1 888 232 4444 (USA & Canada)
phone: 250 383 6864 ♦ fax: 812 355 4082

Previously Published in Canada by:
Help for Headaches
515 Richmond Street, Box 1568
STN B
London, Ontario, Canada
N6A 5M3
phone: 519 434 0008
www.headache-help.org

The scenarios or case studies portrayed and sufferers' names used within this book are fictitious. Any similarity to a name, event or character, or history of any person is entirely coincidental and unintentional.

I am especially indebted to Dr. Joel Saper of the Michigan Headache & Neurological Institute, Ann Arbor, Michigan for his constructive critiques.

Quotes

"My headaches have burdened me for years and I have missed many social functions because of my headaches. People have no idea!"

Audrey - Alberta, Canada

"Thank you for your help. I have looked for information and I must say that I am a bit frustrated. Just having someone that understands is comforting... thanks."

Meme - Nova Scotia, Canada

"Headaches rob you of moments... thereby reducing your quality of life"

Brent - Ontario, Canada

"I would like to thank you for the knowledge and guidance you gave me yesterday. I've been trying to get guidance like that for two and a half years so it gave me some realistic hope."

Tom - Ontario, Canada

Acknowledgements

I would like to express my heart-felt thanks to the numerous headache professionals who gave me insights into the making of this book. Without their expertise this book would have not been possible. Many of these physicians and pharmacists have reviewed articles or have contributed sections.

Thanks to my family (Richard, Karen, Marilyn, John) and to my good friends (Carmen, Saranda, Sadie, Donna,) for their patience as I went on and on about what a global burden headache places on literally billions of people. I would also like to thank numerous other volunteers.

A special thank you to my friend and president Saranda, for her countless hours of volunteer work.

Thanks to Heidi and the team at Chameleon Creative: www.chameleoncreative.com.

Also a special thank you to Michelle at MLS Graphic Design: www.mlsgraphicdesign.ca.

I also thank Merv for his volunteer time.

My wish is that this book will inspire other writers to address the gigantic problem of headache and migraine!

Thanks to Headache Network Canada, The World Headache Alliance and the Canadian Headache Society for their encouragement, and letters of support!

BL

Intentions

This book is intended for educational purposes only and is in no way responsible for your overall well-being. The intent of this book is to provide research and information regarding a very misunderstood health topic.

Please visit our charity website at www.headache-help.org for further information and for order details.

The doctors mentioned herein are given credit for their knowledge but they do not assume liability in any way. Their sole purpose is to educate and to assist you in better understanding headaches so that you can sort out with your own physician or health care professional, what works best for you.

Any similiarities in case illustrations to a real person, living or deceased is purely coincidental.

Preface

This book is all about headaches and migraines. If you are one of the unlucky millions of Canadians who suffer from bad headaches, you are probably saying to yourself, "I can relate".

Headache is one of the most common complaints to mankind, yet little is known about its complexity. It is understandable that the sufferer gets confused with the dizzying array of treatments available.

Headaches are often scoffed at, ridiculed, and have become the topic for endless jokes. By their sheer invisible nature it is no wonder they have been tied to folklore and have said to occupy the minds of demons. Of course this is completely untrue!

Headache is a valid biological disorder that is aggravated by many triggers including certain foods, heredity, some hormonal factors, environmental issues, the stress response, medication overuse, etc. Perhaps it is faire to say that millions of unfortunate headache sufferers are "headache-prone", and that is often linked to heredity. Finding and isolating your trigger and using trigger-avoidance techniques may help you to avoid your next attack.

Stressors are everywhere in today's society and having a headache while under stress seems completely normal for some. On the contrary, millions of people live under tremendous stress every day and many never get headaches. Why is that?

This book is intended for headache sufferers and the professionals who treat them, written in everyday language. As an author and researcher I have never encountered a valid medical disorder so misunderstood and innaccurately diagnosed.

My goal is to bring to the surface a very misunderstood public health topic and to shine a light on it, opening it up to the general public and headache neurologists for discussion in an open, candid, forthright fashion.

Headache sufferers sometimes drift from doctor to doctor, at times clog emergency rooms, some seek out alternative methods that are useless and untested. Some may become alienated from the medical profession and sometimes never improve, or even worsen at times.

Your quality of life is at stake and I encourage you to be an informed patient so that you can be a part of the "finding what works" equation. So the next time someone tries to figure out why you have this awful headache, you candidly reply, "because I am headache-prone"!

BL

Why This Book was Written

The Origin of my own Headache Story and what inspired 'Help for Headaches'; then 'Headaches That Persist'.

The year was 1994 and while most were enjoying the heightened mood during the holiday season, I was experiencing excruciating headaches. These headaches were so terrible that they interrupted my sleep on a nightly basis.

I had tried everything including nerve blocks, oxygen by face mask and even surgery. Initially some relief was achieved (which only added to the confusion), but total relief was not possible.

I travelled great distances at my own expense in search of a cure, or at least some form of consistent relief.

One day, at my breaking point, I went to Dr. Joel Saper's headache centre in Ann Arbor, Michigan, the Michigan Headache & Neurological Institute.

Due to my headache severity, I was immediately admitted to their inpatient program at Chelsea Community Hospital. I can picture it as if it was yesterday - they had an entire hospital wing devoted to treatment of chronic headaches and migraines. Visit their website: www.mhni.com to learn more about the facility.

After years of searching, my severe headaches finally stopped completely - I had finally found an inpatient program that relieved my pain.

Other disorders receive extensive discussion and large amounts of research dollars, but headache remains much of a mystery, even to some of the very professionals trained to treat them. It is no wonder why sufferers feel a sense of apathy or confusion, when conditions like diabetes, according to the Migraine Trust in England, receive a much higher contribution amount from funders.

I am an advocate of inpatient programs, as often intravenous medications are needed to stop the cyclical nature of many headache types.

A 'headache specialist' team approach is needed to pinpoint everything that is going on. We are addressing neurology, psychology, lifestyle, diet, exercise, alternatives, and more. Canada, as of the writing of this book, does not have an inpatient program. Sufferers must still frequent hospital emergency rooms when things get bad. Many headache disorders can be treated successfully by a physician or neurologist on an out-patient basis.

Ask yourself how many times have you tried (unsuccessfully) to locate relief? Have you given that physician and/or medication a chance to work? How many dollars have you spent on over-the-counter remedies, or travel expenses to appointments? Have you done your part in being a proactive patient by reading recommended articles?

I caution the reader not to compare treatments as there are hundreds of headache categories, each with many treatment choices. With so many treatment options it is easy to see why things can become blurred.

I close by cautioning readers that there is a lot of redundant material on the Internet. You will find a large amount of information, much of which is generic. Take your headache pattern seriously. This is the first step!

I truly hope Canada is able to develop an inpatient program, for those that need one!

Brent Lucas

Neurologist Contributors & Reviewers Headache Specialty

Judith Abdalla, M.D., FRCPC
Neurologist - headache specialty
London, Ontario, Canada

American Council for Headache Education (ACHE)
American National Non-Profit
Headaches and Migraines
Mount Royal, New Jersey
www.achenet.org

David Biondi, D.O. Neurologist
Massachusetts General Hospital
Boston, Massachusetts

Dr. Werner J. Becker, MD, FRCPC (neurol)
Professor, Dept of Clinical Neurosciences
Faculty of Medicine
University of Calgary
Calgary, Alberta, Canada.

Barbaranne Branca, PhD, ABPN, DABFE, DABFM
Neuropsychologist - Headache Specialty
Michigan Headache & Neurological Institute
Ann Arbor, Michigan

Paul E. Cooper, M.D., FRCPC Neurology
Special Interest in Headache
London Health Sciences Centre - University Hospital
London, Ontario, Canada

Ian Finkelstein, Msc, M.D., DAAPM
Board Certified, Pain Management
Toronto Headache and Pain Clinic
Toronto, Ontario, Canada

Marek Gawel, MB, Bch, FRCPC
Associate Professor of Medicine, University of Toronto
Staff: Sunnybrook Health Sciences Centre
Woman's College Hospital
Rouge Valley Health System
Special Interest in Headache
Toronto, Ontario, Canada

Rose Giammarco, M.D., FRCPC
Neurologist Headache Specialty
McMaster University
Assistant Clinical Professor
Hamilton Headache Clinic
Hamilton, Ontario, Canada

Robert L.Hamel, M.M., P.A.-C
Physician's Assistant - Program Director
Specialty in Inpatient Hospitalization Services
Michigan Headache & Neurological Institute
Ann Arbor, Michigan

Headache Network Canada (HNC)
Canadian, Web-based, Non-Profit Organization
Headaches and Migraines
Toronto, Ontario, Canada
www.headachenetwork.ca

Help for Headaches (HFH)
Brent Lucas, BA
Ontario Non-Profit
Headache and Migraine Education
London, Ontario, Canada
www.headache-help.org

Alvin Lake III, PhD
Head of Psychology
Michigan Headache & Neurological Institute
Ann Arbor, Michigan

Christine Lay, M.D., FRCP
Board Certified in Neurology and Headache
Director, Woman's College Hospital Centre For Headache
University of Toronto - 76 Greenville St., Ste E 571
Toronto, Ontario, Canada M5S 1B2
Tel: 416.323.6400 x6136

Alexander Mauskop, MD., FAAN,
Board-certified in Neurology and Headache Medicine
Interest in Alternatives
New York Headache Center
30 East 76 Street
New York, New York 10021
Tel: 212.794.3550 - www.NYHeadache.com
Migralex - A New Generation of Headache Relief - Find it at
www.migralex.com

The Migraine Trust
England Headache and Migraine Research
55-56 Russell Square, 2nd Floor,
London, EnglandWC1B 4HP
Tel: 020 7436 1336 Fax: 020 7436 2880
www.migrainetrust.org

Lawrence Robbins, M.D., FACPC
Neurologist - Headache Specialty
Robbins Headache Clinic
Northbrook, Illinois

Joel Saper, M.D., F.A.C.P., F.A.A.N.
Neurologist - Headache specialty
Michigan Headache & Neurological Institute
Ann Arbor, Michigan

Gary Shapero, M.D.
The Shapero Markham Headache and Pain Treatment Centre
10 Unionville Gate, Suite 301
Unionville, Ontario, Canada
L3R 0W7

Fred Sheftell, M.D.
Director and Founder
The New England Center for Headache
Stamford, Connecticut

Stephen Silberstein, M.D., FACPC
Neurologist - Headache Specialty
Germantown Hospital and Medical Center
Jefferson Headache Center
Philadelphia, Pennsylvania

Seymour Solomon, M.D.,
Director Emeritus
Professor of Neurology
Albert Einstein College of Medicine
Montefiore Medical Center
Bronx, New York

Valerie South, R.N.
Neuroscience Nurse
Headache Specialty
Toronto, Ontario, Canada

World Headache Alliance (WHA)
World Non-Profit
Burden of Headache Disorders - Advocacy
London, United Kingdom
www.w-h-a.org

Irene Worthington, R.Ph, B.Sc.Phm
Pharmacist
Headache Network Canada
Toronto, Ontario, Canada

Headaches That Persist

Table of Contents

Chapter 5

Chapter 6

Chapter 7

Chapter 8

Chapter 9

Chapter 10

1

Is it a Migraine or Bad Headache, What Causes a Headache, Prevalence of Headaches, Effects on Society

Understanding your Condition and the Enormous Indirect Costs we all Absorb

Headaches are elusive, sometimes poorly understood by some professionals, and can be lessened or worsened by a number of behavioural and lifestyle factors. It is important to know what influences affect you negatively and positively.

Most sufferers wait months to see a physician as our current medical system is under-funded. Consequently, quality of life deteriorates and the headache sufferers lose their ability to contribute to their family and workplace is heavily impacted. See Chapter 6 - Self-help Strategies, Home Remedies and Workplace Issues.

The same can be true for any condition. But dealing with headaches - from the sufferer's point of view - brings with it a sense of apathy which unfortunately most physicians or health care professionals are left to address.

Reading this book will not only make the sufferer a more informed patient but it will describe issues such as headache causes, prevalence, costs, categories and rare headache types, preventative medicines, abortive medicines, alternatives, self-help strategies, home remedies, workplaces issues, triggers, role of caffeine, tests, emergency room treatments, persons with a disability, chronic daily headache, hormonal factors for women, children, adolescents, people over 50, travel and holidays, preparing for your appointment, diaries, record keeping, and drawing from headache resources.

Is It a Migraine or a Bad Headache?

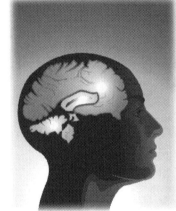

by Brent Lucas, BA – Director, Help for Headaches, London, Canada. Reviewed by Irene Worthington, Pharmacist, Headache Network Canada, Toronto, Canada and Dr. Marek Gawel, MD, Headache Neurologist, Headache Network Canada, Toronto, Canada

Background on "the problem"

Headaches are as old as mankind, yet they continue to confuse many sufferers and even some of the very professionals that are trained to treat them.

When sufferers focus on locating a cure for their headache, they often lose sight of the fact that many treatments both medicinal and holistic, were designed to "reduce" the sensation of the pain experienced, and possibly associated symptoms such as nausea and sensitivity to light and sound. Sufferers can drift from doctor to doctor, occasionally clog emergency rooms, and sometimes seek out ad hoc remedies that are not thoroughly tested, which can be expensive and are often ineffective. There is so much information on migraines and headaches – where should you look?

A headache sufferer can easily locate numerous websites that offer useful information describing the ailment. Be cautious of reading material that describes a migraine but offers little insight into the many types of headaches that exist. Your physician is the best person to point you in the right direction.

Our provincial charity on headaches, dealing mainly with Ontario, is called Help for Headaches. (www.headache-help.org) Help for Headaches is a member of the World Headache Alliance and the Canadian Pain Society.

Headache Network Canada (www.headachenetwork.ca) reaches out to sufferers Canada-wide. Both organizations are registered charities and offer a wealth of free information online.

If a headache sufferer requires inpatient hospitalization, there are American headache centres that offer that service, usually at a significant cost. Canada at this time, does not have an inpatient program exclusively for headaches. That is not to say that chronic sufferers always need hospitalization or emergency services.

Difference between primary and secondary headaches

Primary headaches such as Migraine, Tension-Type and Cluster Headaches are a disorder in themselves whereas secondary headaches like those resulting from hypoglycemia, head injuries or hypertension are secondary symptoms of other ailments. It is important to recognize a severe headache that comes on very suddenly and is very severe – this may be a sign of stroke or other serious problem.

Please keep in mind that most headache sufferers are often experiencing a migraine or a tension-type headache. (Alexander Mauskop, M.D. New York Headache Centre, New York, NY). Some people who think they are suffering from sinus headache are, in fact, suffering from migraine.

Triggers, Record keeping, Home Remedies, Self-Help Techniques, Over-the-Counter

People need to realize that just because they have isolated a food or weather trigger and use trigger-avoidance for their migraine that it does not guarantee another attack will be avoided. In all likelihood a future attack can sometimes be avoided, but there are no guarantees.

Record keeping is very important as physicians use the features you list to classify and track your headache type, which in turn allows them to recommend a treatment.

Home remedies, self-help techniques and over-the-counter approaches are explained in Chapters 3 & 6. A comprehensive list is found on the Help for Headaches website.

Medications versus Alternatives

A few questions to consider might be:
- What are the person's feelings toward the approach being considered?
- Is their physician aware of all other medications/alternatives? (to avoid problems with contradictions and drug interactions).
- Home remedies? Self-help techniques?
- Check your health plan to see if that treatment is covered
- Fitness and lifestyle may need to be modified
- Botulinum toxin (Botox)

An article by Dr. Rose Giammarco, M.D. Hamilton Headache Clinic, Hamilton, ON, Canada is available on the Help for Headaches website: www.headache-help.org/botox.html

How do I find out what headache type I appear to have? I need to locate a headache neurologist in Canada – where do I look?

In terms of treatment, understanding your headache type can point you in the right direction. Help for Headaches has created a "Headache Types Poster", free to view on our website: www.headache-help.org/headache_poster.html, to assist you in comparing your symptoms. There are 9 headache categories discussing location, frequency and severity of the pain experienced. Categories include migraine with aura, migraine without aura, tension-type headache, cluster headache, chronic daily headache, medication overuse headache, stress and headache, headaches in children, and sinus headache. The poster was thoroughly reviewed by Dr. Christine Lay from Toronto, Canada. The poster project was supported by an unrestricted educational grant from Merck Frosst Canada Ltd.

If you require more information and need to locate a headache neurologist in Canada please refer to the "find-a-headache-doctor" link on our website: www.headache-help.org/find_ha_dr.html. There are many physicians qualified to treat migraines or headache but this page lists Canada's top headache neurologists.

Learning your symptoms will always be the single best way of helping yourself.

Patients/sufferers can best help themselves by understanding their "problem" and should work with their doctor to find a treatment that works. Be a proactive and informed patient!

What Causes A Headache?

By Stephen D. Silberstein, M.D. Co-Director, Comprehensive Headache Center, The Germantown Hospital and Medical Center. Philadelphia, PA.

Additional reviews from Christine Lay, MD, FRCP, Director, Women's College Hospital Centre For Headache, Toronto ON, Canada

You may say, "I know what causes my headaches." Staying up late or drinking too much coffee will bring on a headache every time. But a trigger is not the same as a cause. Aged cheese, cigarette smoke, alcohol, excessive caffeine, bright sunlight, disrupted sleep patterns, and many other factors can trigger some migraines in headache prone patients. However, even a known trigger does not always lead to a headache. Therefore, these factors cannot be said to be the cause of headache the way a particular virus is the cause of a head cold or flu. Instead, the nervous system of the headache sufferer is somehow predisposed to respond to these triggers and other stresses with a series of biochemical changes that result in pain and other symptoms of the headache.

Until recently, medical researchers believed that tension-type headache was caused by contraction of muscles of the head and neck, and that migraine headache resulted from the expansion (or dilation) of blood vessels in the brain and scalp. The migraine aura was thought to be due to a constriction of the blood vessels, which preceded the dilation and which reduced blood supply to the eyes and brain. These theories made sense to both physicians and patients, since they counted for the tenderness and the throbbing experienced with these forms of headache, as well as the visual disturbances of aura. However, the vascular (involving blood vessels) theory could not explain many of the other symptoms of migraine, including the mood changes before and after the attack.

The use of new noninvasive technology, such as MRI, PET,

and CT Scans, along with the great advances in understanding the brains biochemistry, have taught us much more about the causes of head pain. As we know, vascular changes may be an important factor in a headache attack, but they are not the whole story nor the root cause. A reduction in brain activity, rather than blood supply, seems to be linked to the migraine aura. Similarly, there is little evidence that muscle contraction causes tension-type headache. Some researchers think that several stages in the complex pain-producing process are similar for these two distinct headache disorders.

The brain and the nerves communicate by means of a special group of chemicals called neurotransmitters. The neurotransmitters are essential for all nervous system functioning, including muscle 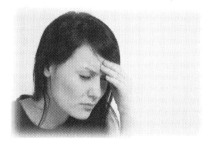 contraction, sensory perception, thought, mood, and awareness of pain. No single neurotransmitter regulates processes so complex as mood and pain perception. Moreover, each neurotransmitter can have multiple roles throughout the brain and nervous system. In migraine, a change in the availability of a particular neurotransmitter called serotonin seems to be the most important single event causing an attack.

Serotonin is known to affect sleep, mood, blood vessel elasticity (constriction & dilation), and contraction of smooth muscles, such as those of the gut. It also regulates the release of another neurotransmitter called substance P, which increases the permeability of capillaries, so that substances leak into surrounding tissue. This local leakage (edema) includes release of an irritating and inflammatory chemical called bradykinin, which stimulates the pain conducting nerves. At the same time, substance P is one of the most powerful facilitators of pain. It make the pain conducting nerve fibers more sensitive to the presence of bradykinin and to substance P itself. This suggests that there are two aspects to the head pain - a "double whammy." The vascular changes maybe a source of pain, but sensitivity to pain has been greatly increased by the action of substance P and bradykinin.

This does not mean that headache sufferers have a "low pain threshold" - a simplistic view of pain that implies personal weakness. Pain perception depends upon the balance of activity of chemicals that decrease or inhibit pain awareness, such as endorphins, and chemicals that increase or facilitate it, such as substance P or bradykinin. If substance P is being released and taken up by the pain-conducting nerves, you cannot help feeling pain any more than you can help hearing a firecracker explode near your ear.

The serotonin theory of migraine also provides an explanation for the mood changes (irritability, depression, or sometimes elation) than many sufferers experience before and/or after an attack. A second neurotransmitter, norepinephrine (noradrenaline), also plays a role in pain perception during migraine. In addition, the female hormone estrogen is known to be involved in migraine, possibly by stimulating prostaglandins, which also cause blood vessels to constrict and dilate. (See Chapter 10 - Women's Issue, Pregnancy & Oral Contraceptives)

Theories are useful. The serotonin theory of migraine, however incomplete it may be, has helped explain how some classes of migraine medication work (such as antidepressants), and has guided efforts to develop more effective ones. Sumatriptan (Imitrex) was designed to have a specific effect on part of the serotonin system. DHE (dihydroergotomine), another headache drug, has also been shown to affect the serotonin system. Sumatriptan's and DHE's success in treating migraine and their usefulness for other types of headache give us important clues to refining our theories of headache. In turn, a more accurate and complete theory can direct the design of more effective medications with fewer side effects.■

Prevalence of Headache

Statistics vary according to country and more importantly physician or researcher, but the following statistics are meant to give you an idea about the prevalence of headache.

- Migraine affects 18% of women, 6% of men and 3% of children. It is a global ailment that touches all races, cultures, personality types and income levels.

- Headache costs our Canadian economy $20 per second (Giammarco, 2006)

- It is estimated that 3.4 million Canadian adults suffer from migraine (Merck Frosst Canada, 2007)

- Over 500 million dollars are lost each year due to worker absenteeism in Canada due to migraine (World Headache Alliance, 2007)

- Chronic Daily Headache affects 3-5% of the population. (American Headache Society, 2007)

- Children who suffer headaches - 10%,   adolescents - 28%, (Robbins, 2006)

- In the US - $2,631. per patient - indirect headache costs (Robbins, 2006)

- In the US - $394. per patient - direct headache costs (Robbins, 2006)

- Approximately 3/4 of migraine sufferers are female (World Headache Alliance, 2007)

- Time spent teaching about headache in undergraduate medical schools amounts to less than 1 hour over 5 years of training as of 1999. (MacGregor, 1999)

- Worldwide, it is estimated that 5,800 million people have first hand experience of the recurrent sick headaches which characterize migraine (Astra Zeneca Canada)

- Migraine is more prevalent in the under-fifties age group - see Chapter 11 - People Over 50 - in fact, nearly 3/4 of adult sufferers are less than forty-five years old (GlaxoSmithKline Canada)

- Migraine is the most common neurological condition in the developed world. It is more prevalent than diabetes, epilepsy and asthma combined (The Migraine Trust, England)

- Migraine is ranked as one of the most disabling illnesses by the World Health Organization (WHO)

Effects on Society

As you can see by the earlier section on "prevalence" - headache is devastating to the financial workings of a society. Without some proper facts to guide you through the murky waters of medical science, it can get expensive and choosing a treatment that is right for you can be very difficult.

When a person is "headache-prone" their quality of life deteriorates and they are often scoffed at or become the topic of jokes at parties. When you are susceptible to frequent headache or migraine attacks you learn what you can manage and to pick your battles.

No one knows the devastation that chronic pain can bring to your life more than your spouse who lives it with you. Even though he or she can physically see your eyes well up in pain, or watch you furrow your brow, or bang your head on the wall (cluster headaches), he or she still does not seem to understand, and asks you why "something can't be done?" Your spouse or partner may even sometimes think you are bringing the headache upon yourself.

Headache brings with it such difficulty and devastation that it is often ridiculed at parties. It is sometimes dismissed by some medical professionals which no doubt leaves the sufferer feeling perplexed, confused and distraught.

Headache-prone people tend to isolate themselves which is diametrically oppposed to what is best for them. We know behaviour plays such a pivotal role in overall scheme of things, when a proper diagnosis is made, it makes sense to practice good social networking skills and work on the problem together. Be sure to mention any fitness exercise programs or any headache support groups to your doctor.

Alternatives can be a great way to treat your headaches - (see Chapter 5 - Alternative Treatments & Botox), but a few errors that sufferers make when using alternative methods are:

- they don't mention them to their physician

- they do not get advice on contraindications with any other headache medicines or treatments

- they forget to check their drug coverage plan before they order large amounts

- they switch to alternatives (which are tested less rigorously) from traditional medicines, without doing appropriate research.

- they don't read about potential side effects

Many headache sufferers have been unfairly blamed for their illness for too long. Despite advances in modern medicine, enormous amounts of time and money are wasted on gimmicks which are found to be sadly inadequate. This results in billions of dollars wasted and headache sufferers often become frustrated or angry, and many simply give up the search for an effective treatment plan. A skilled physician will continue to be the best person to help you find relief. Be sure to do your part and walk into your appointment with a sound understanding of your headaches and how your body reacts to them.

Editor's note:

This book is intended for educational purposes only and is not intended to replace a physician's advice or treatment. Learning your individual symptoms will always be the single most important thing that you can do for yourself.

2

Headache Categories,
Rare Headache Types, Stroke

Understanding Your Condition is the First Step

There is so much to know concerning headaches that we can often become discouraged. A thorough and complete understanding of your headache pattern or ailment will certainly assist in the sorting out stage.

Coming prepared with good record keeping (see Diary - Chapter 13 - How To Prepare for your Physician's Appointment?) it will assist in narrowing the search for an effective treatment. All treatments are effective but many may not be suitable for you. I understand your frustration of finding a cure. However, in defense of a General Practioner's schedule many are just too busy to devote additional time to this complex disorder. If additional or aggressive treatments are sought by the headache sufferer, consider consulting with a headache neurologist or a physician with an interest in this field of neurology or headaches.

Below I have listed a number of categories for you to compare. Sometimes you will notice how you have a few features of one category mixed with a few symptoms of another category. These are clues to mention to your doctor in case you have multiple headache conditions.

The work you do ahead of time and in between appointments can often lead to answers surfacing with tips for techniques and treatments.

Ask yourself the following questions:

- Are my headaches beginning for the first time?

- Are they predictable - eg. time of day, location, triggers, storm fronts, hormonal?

- Are there family histories of migraines or headaches? Are they hereditary?

- Am I using any non-pharmacological techniques? Vitamins? Herbs? (Please tell your physician)

- What makes them worse? What makes them better?

- Do they respond to Medications? Alternatives? Self-Help Techniques?

- What am I taking now for them? (Over-the-Counter remedies, Triptans, Motrin, Tylenol, Aspirin, Advil?)

Migraine without Aura (Common Migraine)

Usually this is a one-sided very painful headache, which can last 4-72 hours. Migraine without Aura is severe in intensity and is often (75%) seen in women who are usually in their child-bearing years. It is a pulsating or throbbing sensation of pain. 70% of sufferers often have a family history of migraine. Sometimes common migraines can be brought on by a food, weather or stress "trigger"- see Triggers – Chapter7 - but a trigger is not the same thing as a cause. Common migraine is a biological problem that can affect anyone. Changes in brain chemistry produce neurological and physical symptoms. These symptoms and sensations are important to learn and record as that is how physicians diagnose migraine. Due to a broad range of symptoms among sufferers, it is recommended to consult with a headache physician and a pharmacist on a regular basis. These migraine headaches are often mild to moderate in pain severity, and they often present themselves as severe.

Migraine with Aura (Classic Migraine)

Migraines that are preceded by neurological warning signs are often referred to as Migraine with Aura. The aura that suggests that the migraine is on its way is characterized by symptoms such as flickering lights or black spots in the field of vision. Wavy, zig-zag lines characteristic of a spider web can be present in the field of vision also. Occasional numbness on one side of the face or hand can also occur, suggestive of an aura. The headache pain following the aura is typically a one-sided headache with a throbbing or pounding sensation of pain, often signifying migraine with aura. The aura, a warning sign that this category of migraine is on its way, is experienced in about 15% - 19% of people suffering with migraines. They experience changes in brain function that can seem strange or bizarre. It is common for sufferers to experience neurological symptoms such as difficulty speaking, imbalance, vertigo, loss of consciousness and paralysis or numbness. Visual symptoms such as a blind spot in the field of vision are the most common features. Sometimes the headache associated with this migraine type might be very mild or even absent. These types of migraines can be mild to moderate in severity and are often severe in their pain quality. Migraine with aura is not completely understood, but there are effective medical treatments available. Consult with a physician and sometimes with a neurologist with interest in headaches.

Tension-Type Headache

Tension-type headaches are the most common type of headache and are found in over three-quarters of headache patterns. They have been reported as a headache condition felt on both sides of the head and are described as tight, non-pulsating, pressing or squeezing band-like pain. As muscles tighten in the head and

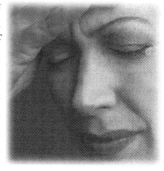

neck and blood vessels in the head expand, headache pain is often experienced on the forehead or on both sides of the head. The pain can be experienced as a "tight-hat" sensation or a pressing, squeezing sensation of pain. The location of the pain often moves, covering the temples, crown, front or back of the head and neck. Unlike migraine, this headache type is usually not aggravated by daily routine. Some experts argue that tension-type headache pain is actually a variant of migraine pain. Tension headaches were once labeled as a psychological cause for head pain by some sufferers. Today we know changes in brain chemistry often induce a Tension-Type Headache. Almost everyone suffers occasionally from muscle contraction headaches (an older name once used). In its chronic form it represents a painful annoyance, and is referred to as a Chronic Tension-Type Headache which can be very stubborn to treat for both the sufferer and by a headache physician. For more information on Chronic Tension-Type Headache see the listing mentioned later in this chapter and consult the index at the end of this publication. Care should be taken not to over-medicate and cause Medication Overuse Headaches known formerly as Rebound Headaches.

Cluster Headache

A "Cluster Headache" is arguably the most sinister of all headache types. Unlike migraine which is largely a female problem, almost all cluster headache sufferers are male. One-sided headache attacks come in bouts or a series of pain, which is why these headache types are called "clusters". A teary eye on the affected side is common as well as a drooped eyelid on the affected side. Also, running of the nose or nasal discharge has been recorded. The pain duration of cluster headache is typically 1-3 hours, whereas migraine is generally 7 hours or more. Cluster headache sufferers are in so much pain that sufferers typically bang their heads on the wall, in total frustration. Direct oxygen has been an effective relief for some sufferers as well as many other medications. For some extreme cases even surgery is recommended by a physician. Often medications are used to avert an attack or to prevent further subsequent attacks. A number of medications can be used to successfully treat cluster headache. For addition resources go to www.clusterheadaches.com

A very similar headache condition to cluster and sometimes easily confused is a headache condition know as Hemicrania Continua - see Chronic Daily Headache article - Chapter 9.

In cluster headache both the episodic type (described above) and the chronic cluster headache type (described next) are listed. In the episodic form there are generally cycles or bouts of recurring headaches that occur for 3-4 months at a time, sometimes longer or shorter, and then go into a remission (holiday) in which there will be no headaches present for months, or longer.

The chronic form may start as a chronic headache, without any prolonged period of headache absence, or it may evolve from the seasonal, episodic type. Chronic cluster headache is fully explained below.

Chronic Cluster Headaches

Occasionally, cluster headaches evolve into a rare headache known as Chronic Cluster Headaches. Unlike regular cluster headaches that typically take a holiday - the chronic form is just that - chronic. Most headache books do not even carry this term in their index, it is so rare. Chronic cluster headaches can, at times, be mistaken for other pain conditions, but the following checklist may aid you in determining if you have this very painful condition.

One headache neurologist in Michigan uses this checklist:

- Almost always one-sided extremely painful attacks

- Usually focuses in one eye, causing it to tear

- Refuses to take a holiday like regular clusters

- A knife-like sensation of pain usually through one eye

- Have been labeled as "suicide headaches" because the pain is so unbearable.

- Documentation has cited the hypothalamus near the pituitary gland and other regions of the brain, and surrounding areas likely provoke cluster headache or related headache forms. There needs to be further research performed to confirm this.

- Intravenous medications are sometimes an effective treatment choice, and which are administered by a physician in a hospital setting.

Migraine Equivalents

This type of headache can feature neurological symptoms or non-neurological symptoms, such as abdominal pain, vertigo, even emotional outbursts, depression or panic. The word equivalent suggests that sufferers instead of a headache, are having some other equivalent troubling symptom. This condition is much more common in children and can resemble stroke-like symptoms which are a numbness or tingling on the arm - absent of any headache which can often be referred to as a migraine equivalent. Also younger children often complain of an upset stomach - absent of any headache. This can often also be a migraine equivalent. Once the child has thrown up, there is often an easing up and relief of the headache symptoms. This headache type is experienced in the stomach which just happens to be the location where a lot of the neurotransmitter serotonin is located.

Sinus Headache

True sinus headache will show up on an x-ray and the sufferer will experience a yellow-green discharge from their nasal area. Migraine headaches are often confused as sinus headaches as the pain of migraine often gets referred to areas of the face, including the ear, nose and jaw, at times. Please see the article on www.headache-help.org/free articles - sinus headache, for further explanations and treatments.

Menstrual Migraine

Migraines which usually come at the time when a woman is having her monthly menstrual cycle are often called Menstrual Migraines. It is clearly evident that the fall of the female hormone of estrogen may be what incites the acute headache in a menstrual migraine, somewhat like in estrogen withdrawl. Much has been written about the connection between estrogen, progesterone and serotonin and there is also a free article at our website www.headache-help.org with an article on "Woman's Issues & Headache". It is no secret that women in their child-bearing years make up 70% - 80% of migraine sufferers, hypothesized largely, because of the hormonal connection. An endocrinologist with interest in migraine would be suggested as a possible source for answers. A female neurologist with great insight into this complex area is also recommended.

Chronic Daily Headache

Chronic Daily Headache is a relatively new term that usually means features of a migraine headache, with additional features of a tension-type headache. In the past, the term mixed headache has been used to describe this headache type. Researchers and scientists all agree that excessive medication overuse is frequently a factor in the sufferer acquiring Chronic Daily Headaches.

Chronic Daily Headache is an umbrella term under which 4 categories of headaches exists, which include; chronic migraine/transformed migraine, chronic tension-type headache, hemicrania continua and new daily persistent headache. Please refer to a comprehensive article on CDH in chapter 9.

It is important to note that Chronic Daily Headache is the umbrella term for the classification of chronic migraine. This still often remains very confusing to physicians and it is important to remember that many headache types can occur daily or almost daily for many sufferers.

The above headache categories were reviewed by Dr. Joel Saper, Michigan Headache & Neurological Institute, Ann Arbor, Michigan.

Rare or Unusual Headache Conditions
My Headaches are Rare and it's Hard to Find Information on Them!

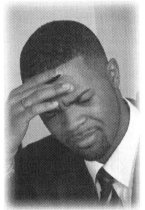

"I searched high and low and cannot seem to find credible information on my specific rare headache type".

Below I have listed a few unusual headache conditions for which information is hard to find.

It is important to learn the features of your condition. That is how your doctor or health professional arrives at a diagnosis, which then narrows the search for an effective treatment choice.

Hot Dog Headache

Nitrites that are often found in hotdogs, gives this rare headache the name "hot dog headache". Nitrites are powerful triggers and can cause blood vessels to swell, thus causing a headache.

The nitrites found in hotdogs are responsible for this headache type. It is important to understand that any sandwhich or processed meat that contains nitrites can also produce a 'hot dog headache'.

If nitrites were your headache trigger the easiest solution would be to use trigger-avoidance whenever possible.

Ice Cream Headache

An ice cream headache can also be referred to as a cold stimulus headache. At times, with headache sufferers, putting cold ice cream on the roof of your tongue can produce a headache.

The same term is used for a headache arising from a cold object in the back of the throat near or by the soft palate. Ice cream is simply one food item that can cause this headache type.

Again, avoiding that trigger would be the fastest solution to living a pain-free life.

Headache After Head Injuries (Post Traumatic Headache)

Not necessarily a benign headache condition, Headache after Head Injuries can often commence after a fall or injury thus giving it the name Post Traumatic Headache. Once the concussion or head injury heals often the headaches will disappear. Typically, the sufferer will experience a dull, diffuse pain felt on both sides of the head.

In many cases of post traumatic headache the neck is more significantly involved and may be the cause of the sustaining headache. The headache may be chronic, and then the term 'chronic post-traumatic headache' is used, when that evolves.

As there is a full article on Headaches After Head Injuries - see Chapter 8 - I will not go into detail about it here.

Temporomandibular Joint Pain (TMJ)

The "hinge" that connects the upper jaw to the lower jaw is called the TMJ or temporomandibular joint. The disc on the TMJ can produce pain to the jaw area. There has been much controversy in the literature about the TMJ as we know migraine headache pain can also be referred to the jaw area. Many headache sufferers have had dental surgeries unnecessarily, although TMJ dysfunction does exist. Please consult with a headache neurologist before consenting to any jaw surgery. In the US go to www.tmj. org for scientific help, and also see - Chapter 14 - Additional Resources to help you.

Hypnic Headache

Hypnic headache is a rare, distinctive nocturnal headache disorder that affects elderly men and women (usually after age 60). The attacks usually occur on both sides, but one-sided pain has been reported (Gould, 1997). The pain is throbbing in quality and occurs 2-4 hours after night-time sleep onset, although attacks after daytime napping are reported (Dodick, 1998). It is usually a short-lived attack with a duration ranging between 15 minutes to 3 hours. Generally, there is an absence of associated autonomic features, although nausea may be present. Hypnic headaches characteristically respond to lithium carbonate (300-600 mg. at h.s.), although caffeine (Dodick, 1998) and indomethacin are also reported to help (Ivanez, 1998). Both genders are affected; however, in Dodick's recent large series, 84% of cases were women. It is generally considered a benign disorder (Gould, 1997; Mosek, 1997; Newman, 1991; Raskin, 1997). At this time, a relationship to cluster headache has not been established. However, the responsiveness to lithium, the periodicity of the attacks, and their nocturnal relationship do raise the question, since these are also features of cluster headache. Raskin (1997) suggests the possibility of disturbances of the "biological clock," which are serotoninergically modulated. Lithium enhances serotoninergic neurotransmission nocturnal headaches, very similar to what have been called hypnic headaches, may occur from other headache conditions, including nocturnal hypoglycemia (low blood sugar), neck disturbances (such as arthritis and degenerative cervical disturbances), withdrawal from caffeine or other substances, and many others. While hypnic headache is one of the causes, the reader should be aware that many other headaches occur at night, not the least of which are migraine and cluster headache.

What is hemiplegic migraine?

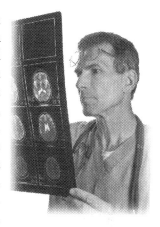

A rare but frightening condition is the hemiplegic migraine which is a typical migraine headache associated with complete or partial paralysis on one side of the body. The paralysis can last from hours to days in duration, followed by a full recovery of strength. An attack of hemiplegic migraine can be triggered by minor head trauma such as that experienced in sports, or by other typical migraine triggers. Hemiplegic migraine attacks can occur in young children and may persist into adulthood. It may be a hereditary condition.

Hypnic Headache and Hemiplegic Migraine descriptions were reprinted with permission from the MHNI website at www. mhni.com – reviewed by Dr. Joel Saper, Michigan Headache & Neurological Institute, Ann Arbor, Michigan. Dr. Joel Saper further reviewed the section on rare headaches.

It is important to mention here that there are many types of rare headaches, and space does not permit me to list them all.

Migraine and stroke – is there a link?
There is considerable interest in the relationship between migraine and stroke.

What is a stroke?

A stroke occurs when part of your brain is deprived of its blood supply. There are two main types of stroke, one of which is suggested to have a link with certain types of migraine.

Migraine affects three times the number of women than men. The incidence of stroke in men is twice that of women. Several studies have shown that the risk of ischemic stroke was increased in women aged under 35 to 45 years old who had migraine with or without aura and was exacerbated by oral contraceptive use, smoking and high blood pressure. Ischemic means a reduced blood and oxygen supply sometimes due to a clot. The other type of stroke is a haemorrhagic stroke, which is where a damaged or weakened artery bleeds into nearby tissue. This type of stroke is not linked with migraine.

Whilst several studies have shown a relative increased risk of stroke in young women with migraine compared to people without migraine, in absolute terms this risk remains extremely small since stroke is rare in young people.

Is there a risk of stroke during a migraine attack?

Understandably, some people are afraid that their migraine is a symptom of a stroke and others worry that they are more at risk of a stroke during a migraine attack. There is little evidence to suggest that a stroke is more likely to occur during a migraine attack than at another time. Migraine is common. In some people migraine and stroke appear together but the nature of the casual relationship, if any, is difficult to establish firmly. Migrainous infarction is the term given to an ischemic stroke occurring during a migraine attack. In this condition aura symptoms are prolonged, and ischemic stroke is confirmed by being shown in a brain scan. However, research suggests that such a stroke would be independent of the migraine attack. It is also possible for a person to have a stroke but for this to have been mistaken for a migraine attack. The migraine aura can mimic transient ischemic attacks

(TIAs). Conversely, in stroke, headache similar to migraine may occur.

What do the statistics show about migraine and stroke?

Numerous studies have been devoted to migraine as a risk factor for ischemic stroke. The majority showed a statistically significant relationship between migraine and ischemic stroke in women aged under 45 years. The increase in risk is more marked for migraine with aura than in migraine without aura, for which there is less evidence. The risk is more than tripled by smoking and quadrupled by oral contraceptive pill use. The triple combination of migraine, oral contraceptive pill use and smoking further increases the risk. Here oral contraceptive refers to combination estrogen/progesterone pills with relatively high doses of estrogen. A review published in 1997 looked at some of the studies in terms of 100,000 women per year. It was suggested that in women under age 35:

- those who do not have migraine and do not take the pill (i.e. the background risk): 1.3 per 100,000 women per year are at risk of stroke

- those who have migraine without aura but don't take the pill: 4 per 100,000 women per year at risk of stroke -those who have migraine with aura but don't take the pill: 8 per 100,000 women per year are at risk of stroke

- those who don't have migraine and take the pill: 5 per 100,000 women per year at risk of stroke

- those who have migraine with aura and take the pill: 28 per 100,000 women per year at risk of stroke

- those who have migraine without aura and take the pill: 14 per 100,000 women per year are at risk of stroke

To put this into context, other studies have suggested that 8 per 100,000 women per year might die in a road accident and 167 per 100,000 women per year might die from a smoking related problem.

A study in America in 2004, called the Women's Health Study, looked at 39,754 female health professionals. During the 9 years of the study there were 309 ischemic strokes in the total population in the study, so there was a total incidence of 8 ischemic strokes per 100,000 women (0.008%). This includes women with and without migraine aura, so it can be seen that although the relative risk is seemingly high, the actual risk is extremely small. This study confirmed previous studies suggesting that the association between migraine aura and stroke risk was greater in younger than in older women (in this case meaning women under age 55). The higher risk with aura will also include those who have other medical conditions that increase the risk of stroke and which can be associated with aura symptoms rather than true migraine aura. These conditions include some blood clotting disorders and heart conditions. The diagnosis of migraine and migraine aura was self-reported so is subject to bias (that is, there was not an objective person to make the diagnosis).

Why should young women with migraine with aura be at an increased risk of stroke?

The mechanism of the increased risk of ischemic stroke in young women with migraine remains unknown. It does not seem to be due to an increase in conventional risk factors such as diabetes, high blood pressure and raised cholesterol levels. There are frequent reports of discoveries of differences between people with and without migraine, for example, the recent attention given to patent foramen ovale (PFO) or hole in the heart in patients with migraine with aura. However, these characteristics are not consistently found in people with migraine compared with people without migraine and they show no sex difference, so that they cannot explain why the increased risk of ischemic stroke in migraine is statistically significant in young women.

Some recent studies suggest that aura is associated with adverse cardiovascular risk profile and prothrombotic factors (tendency of blood to clot). Research is continuing to look into this area in the hope of discovering more about the complex relationship between migraine with aura and ischemic stroke, and any underlying vascular differences between people with and without migraine.

What are the implications?

Whatever the underlying mechanism, the practical implications of the increased ischemic stroke risk in young women with migraine with aura are relatively clear: when the low absolute risk and its increase by cigarette smoking are taken into account, the first recommendation is not to smoke.

The Faculty of Family Planning and the Family Planning Association guidelines confirm that best practice is to contraindicate the combined contraceptive pill for use by women who have migraine with aura, which is also in line with World Health Organization recommendations. The risk for women with migraine without aura is lower and other risk factors like smoking are far more likely to increase stroke risk than migraine. However, in practice, given the very low absolute risk of stroke in young women, there is no systematic contraindication to oral contraceptive use but rather a firm recommendation for no smoking and for the use of low estrogen or progesterone only pills particularly for women with migraine with aura. It is important that women with migraine who are taking the pill do not decide to suddenly stop taking it without discussing this with their doctor. Being 'at risk' of stroke does not mean dying from a stroke. Around 25% of people who have stroke recover, and another 50% will have a disability after a stroke.

What about older people with migraine?

Migraine is considered to be insignificant as a risk factor for stroke after the age of 50 years. This is because the usual risk factors for ischemic stroke are high blood pressure, obesity, raised blood cholesterol levels, smoking and older age. These factors tend to combine with each other and, with advancing age, the risk of stroke due to migraine becomes insignificant in comparison with the other risk factors.

Migraine with aura stands out as a stroke risk of young women because it affects people before the usual and more significant age-related factors apply. In addition migraine tends to improve in later life.

**ALWAYS CONSULT YOUR DOCTOR BEFORE
TAKING OR CHANGING ANY TREATMENTS.
THIS INFORMATION SHOULD NOT
BE A SUBSTITUTE FOR YOUR DOCTOR'S ADVICE.**

Further reading:
– Silberstein, S., Lipton, R. and Goadsby, P. Headache in clinical practice 2nd edition. London: Martin Dunitz; 2002.
– Dowson, A. Migraine and other headaches: your questions answered. London: Churchill Livingstone; 2003.
– MacGregor, A. Understanding migraine and other headaches. Revised edition. London: Family Doctor Publications in association with the British Medical Association; 2006.
Reprinted with permission from the Migraine Trust in the United Kingdom This article is in larger print on request.

Chronic Paroxysmal Hemicrania

Headache doctors suggest that this condition is a variant of the cluster headache family and it is almost generally exclusive to women. (Women generally in their mid 20's to mid 30's are more susceptible). Better known as CPH, the sufferer generally has 5-20 attacks a day, and they usually last under 15 minutes. They are generally more focused around the eye area (similar to cluster), temple or forehead. They are usually a stabbing, knife-like sensation of pain. A tearing eye may also be experienced. A runny or stuffy nose is sometimes present with CPH.

Medication Treatment of CPH

CPH is almost always relieved by indomethacin (Indocin), an anti-inflammatory medication. If indomethacin does not help, the diagnosis of CPH is in doubt (although it still could be CPH). The dose of indomethacin varies greatly with some patients requiring as little as 25mg per day and others needing 250mg or more. Although the Indocin SR 75mg renders dosing more convenient, the 25 or 50mg capsules, taken throughout the day, may be more effective. Patients may titrate their own dose, for at times the attacks may decrease in severity. Usually, when Indocin is tapered or stopped, the attacks resume, but long term remissions may occur. Indomethacin should be taken with food, as GI upset is very common. Although headache may occur as a side effect of indomethacin, it is not common in patients with preexisting headaches. Cognitive side effects, such as fatigue, lightheadedness, and mood swings, may be a problem with indomethacin. Retinal or corneal problems have been reported with long term use of indomethacin. As with all of the anti-inflammatories, renal and hepatic functions need to be monitored through blood tests. Tachyphylaxis does not usually occur with indomethacin.

Corticosteroids, naproxen, and calcium blockers (verapamil) may provide some benefit, but these have limited usefulness in CPH. Acetazolamide may be of benefit in some patients. The triptans do not appear to be particularly effective for CPH.

Medication section of the CPH article reprinted with permission from www.headachedrugs.com - Robbins Headache Clinic, Northbrook, Illinois. Permission from Dr. Lawrence Robbins, MD.

Occipital Neuralgia or back of the head sharp pain

These headaches are described as a burning, sharp, jabbing sensation of pain at the back of the head. Usually the treating physician administers nerve-block injections at the pain site, which generally helps ease the pain. Occipital neuralgia may also stem from injury, whiplash, or from shingles. Many sufferers who have this condition respond favorably to injection treatment. Occasionally, physical therapy may be helpful.

Chronic Tension-Type Headache

Chronic tension-type Headache (CTTH) is the usual episodic (occasional) tension headache in its chronic form. These chronic headaches can be at times a real challenge to treat. These headaches are daily or almost daily in duration and often sleep disturbances (see www.headache-help.org - free articles - Sleep & Headache) play a contributing factor. Chronic tension-type headaches are often found in women ages 30 to 50 and an over-use of over-the-counter medicines is often a contributing factor. For more on CTTH see Chronic Daily Headache article - Chapter 9.

3

Acute Medicines, Over-The-Counter Remedies & Headaches Due To Disease

How Much is Too Much Medicine and the Risk of Developing "Medication Overuse Headache"

Acute Medicines (or symptomatic or abortive/rescue medicines)

What are Acute Medicines or Abortive Medicines and what are they used for?

The last 15 years have seen the development of numerous "triptan medications" that are designed to specifically stop a migraine headache attack and relieve associated symptoms such as nausea/vomiting and sensitivity to light/sound.

Triptan headache medicines are designed to abort (stop) a headache in process. These medicines chemically resemble serotonin, the neurotransmitter that plays a major role in blood vessel dilation in migraine sufferers. All of the triptan medicines have been shown to be effective for migraine headache attacks but some sufferers respond better to one drug than another (if one medicine does not seem to be working, it may be useful to try another medicine, or even a second one, or a third one for future attacks.)

When a migraine is moderate to severe in intensity, physicians often prescribe abortive or "acute therapy" medicines.

Additionally, analgesics (such as ASA or acetaminophen) and non-steroidal anti-inflammatory drugs (NSAIDS, such as ibuprofen or naproxen) are abortive headache medicines as well. They are effective for mild to moderate migraine headache attacks. They are sometimes used in combination with triptan medicines (there is a combination product available in the U.S. – but not Canada as of the publishing of this book – that contains naproxen and sumatriptan – brand name Treximet.)

Below I have listed most of the available triptan medicines that abort a headache in process. As well, I have included some of the newer "triptans". See online interview at *www.headache-help.org* – homepage - interview graphic - Q# 2 for more information about triptan medicines.

Please speak to your doctor about these medicines and follow your physician's advice. A huge factor we see and hear very often is that sufferers have discontinued a medication because it appears to not be working for them. Always talk to your physician first before discontinuing any medication.

This is a general guide only to be used for educational purposes and should not replace a physician's advice.

Sumatriptan (Imitrex)

Sumatriptan (Imitrex) is the oldest and first triptan medicine to be developed. It is a "migraine-specific" medicine which is intended for use in aborting a migraine in process. The injection works very quickly to stop a migraine headache attack (about 15 minutes). Sumatriptan is an effective acute form of treatment and it comes in a few ways of administering it, such as:

• Oral Tablets or DF tablets (dissolve in stomach)
• Injections (to be administered subcutaneously).
• Nasal spray

> *The nasal spray is often prescribed if vomiting is a factor with the migraine sufferer.*

Zolmitriptan (Zomig)

Zolmitriptan (Zomig), another triptan that is used to abort a migraine headache attack, comes in three forms - a tablet form for absorption in the stomach, a rapid-melt wafer (Rapidmelt) that dissolves in the mouth (but gets absorbed in the stomach) and a nasal spray to bypass the stomach area, where nausea and vomiting occur. The wafer form does not act faster than the regular tablet form – it dissolves in the mouth and is swallowed with saliva, to be absorbed in the stomach. It is a convenient and discrete way of taking migraine medicine while traveling. The nasal spray gets partially absorbed in the nasal passageway and has a very fast onset of action (about 45 minutes).

Rizatriptan (Maxalt)

Rizatriptan (Maxalt) comes in a tablet and wafer (RPD) that dissolves in the mouth to abort a migraine headache attack. The wafer can be very useful if nausea is a factor with the migraine attack. Rizatriptan is also available in a tablet form. Both the tablet and wafer start working in about 1 to 1 ½ hours.

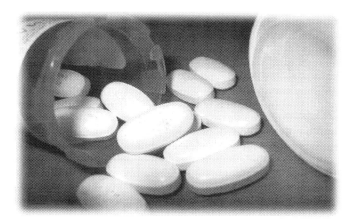

Naratriptan (Amerge)

Naratriptan (Amerge) is a migraine abortive medicine that comes in a tablet form. It can be useful in aborting a migraine in progress. It is usually very well tolerated but it may take up to 3 hours to start working.

Almotriptan (Axert)

Almotriptan (Axert) is a migraine-specific abortive medicine that is fairly new to the triptan family, for stopping a migraine headache attack. It comes in a tablet form and is usually well tolerated. It starts working in about ½ hour to 2 hours.

Eletriptan (Relpax)

Eletriptan (Relpax) is one of the newest additions of acute medicines to emerge. It has been effective in aborting, or stopping, a migraine headache attack. It starts acting in about ½ hour to 1 hour.

Frovatriptan (Frova)

Frovatriptan (Frova) is the newest triptan available in the US, and is now available in Canada. It is a migraine-specific medication that was designed to abort (stop) a migraine headache attack.

Table 1: Migraine Specific Medications and Methods of administration				
Medication	**Tablet**	**Wafer**	**Nasal Spray**	**Injectable**
Naratriptan (Amerge)	✓			
Almotriptan (Axert)	✓			
Sumatriptan (Imitrex)	✓		✓	✓
Rizatriptan (Maxalt)	✓	✓		
Eletriptan (Relpax)	✓			
Zolmitriptan (Zomig)	✓	✓	✓	
Frovatriptan (Frova)	✓			

Reviewed by Irene Worthington, R.Ph., B.Sc.Phm
Drug Information Pharmacist
Sunnybrook Health Sciences Centre, Toronto, Canada

Additional reviews from Dr. Gary Shapero, Markham
Headache & Pain Treatment Centre, Unionville, Ontario, Canada

Ergot Derivatives

Ergot derivatives (such as ergotamine) are older drugs that are sometimes prescribed for migraine sufferers. They are not used very often, as they have many side effects (triptans are preferred). However, dihydroergotamine, in nasal spray form or as an injection (given in hospital usually), has fewer side effects than ergotamine and can be very effective for migraine, especially if it is a prolonged attack. Narcotics (such as codeine) and/or barbiturates (such as butalbital), usually combined with acetaminophen or ASA, are sometimes used, but they have the potential for dependence or addiction, and need to be closely monitored. Remember that all medications produce side effects, so it is very important to openly discuss any medicines (even over-the-counter or herbal products) that are being used to treat headaches. If these medications are taken too often, this can result in chronic headaches (medication overuse headache).

Reviewed by Irene Worthington, R.Ph., B.Sc.Phm
Drug Information Pharmacist

Sunnybrook Health Sciences Centre, Toronto, Canada

Botox (Boutalium Toxin) is an injection that has shown promise in recent years, in stopping a migraine attack. This agent comes in the form of an injection and is actually considered a drug for migraine. Even though Botox is a prophylactic therapy, I mention it briefly here. For a complete explanation on Botox go to: ***www.headache-help.org*** - (button on Botox) or *See online interview (click on interview graphic on website homepage - Q #10 and also see Chapter 5, Botox article.*

Studies are still ongoing to prove its efficiency.

Over-the-Counter Remedies
(that can be purchased without a prescription)

Listed below are a few of the more common Over-the-Counter medicines used for headache, which include:

-Acetaminophen (Tylenol)
-Acetaminophen (Tylenol Extra Strength)
-Ibuprofen (Advil)
-Ibuprofen (Advil Migraine)
-Ibuprofen (Motrin)
-Acetaminophen & ASA & Caffeine (Excedrin)
-Acetaminophen & ASA & Caffeine (Excedrin Extra Strength)
-Aspirin-Free Exedrin
-ASA (Aspirin)
-ASA & Caffeine (Anacin)

Over-the-counter medicines are also effective in mild headache attacks when relaxation techniques, caffeine and alternatives fail to work. Also, triptan therapy is often used in milder attacks. Caution should be exercised when using over-the-counter medicines as these medicines have the potential for misuse *(Medication Overuse Headache - see Chapter 9)*, which is very strong. The headache partially goes away with a regular amount of over-the-counter medicine, thereby making the sufferer believe that they have not taken enough of that product. The cycle of - "more medication needed"- begins. Over-the-Counter medicines are easily purchased at any drug store and they often line the shelves of most supermarkets.

You do not need a prescription for over-the-counter headache medicines.

Again, it is worth mentioning here that Medication Overuse Headache can also be attained from taking too much abortive medicine (see Chapter 9 - Chronic Daily Headache, Fibromyalgia & Chronic Fatigue Syndrome) or from overusing over-the-counter pain relievers for headache. Always follow a physician's advice, especially in regards to dosages and how often these medications can be taken.

I will mention here that Triptan Headache Medicines can cause medication overuse and should be followed from a physician's advice.

Headache Triggers

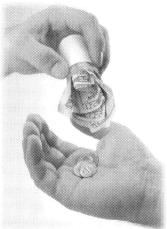

Below I have listed a very brief list of triggers (reprinted with permission from an international headache neurologist), Dr. Lawrence Robbins. I explain "migraine triggers" more thoroughly in Chapter 7 - Headache Triggers, Caffeine and Social Support.

Common Migraine Triggers
- Overwhelming "daily headache"
- Stress, worry, depression, and anger
- Some foods
- Weather and seasonal changes, such as humidity or high heat
- Smoke, perfume, gasoline, paint, organic solvents, and other strong odors
- Hunger
- Fatigue or lack of sleep
- Hormonal factors such as menstruation, birth control pills, pregnancy, menopause, estrogens
- Oversleeping and excessive sleep
- Bright lights, such as glaring artificial lights or bright sunlight
- Head Trauma
- Altitude
- Motion, experienced during car rides or amusement park rides, for example

Please note that identifying your headache trigger and using "trigger-avoidance" is a very powerful way to prevent your next migraine. This is a short list of potential migraine triggers, and a much more comprehensive list can be found on Chapter 7 - Headache Triggers, Caffeine & Social Support.

> (the word "analgesics" comes from
> the Greek word "an", meaning without, and "algos"
> meaning pain)

Headaches Due To Disease
by Judith Anne Abdalla, M.D.,
F.R.C.P. C. Neurology
London, Ontario, Canada

In 1988 The International Headache Society developed a method of classification for headaches as a tool for physicians. Despite some drawbacks it has been very useful. Many different headache types have been named and classified in broad types. The International Headache Society describes the following types of headaches.

Primary Headache Disorders

• Migraine
• Tension-Type Headache
• Cluster Headache
• Chronic Paraxysmal Hemicrania
• Miscellaneous Benign Dysfunctional Headaches such as "ice pick pains", "benign sex headache", "ice cream headache", etc.

Secondary Headaches

• Post Traumatic Headaches   - acute
                              - chronic
• Headaches Associated with Vascular Disorders

- Headaches from other Intracranial Diseases
        -high CFS Pressure
        -tumour
        -pseudotumour
        -hydrocephalus
        -low CSF Pressure
        -infection (Meningitis, etc.)
        -inflammation (Eg. Lupus, Sarcoidosis)
        -other

- Headaches associated with Substances or their withdrawal
- Headaches associated with Systemic (ie. Not head) infections
        -viral
        -bacterial
        -other
- Headaches associated with metabolic disorders such as high altitude, sleep apnea, low blood sugar headache, etc.
- Headaches associated with Disease of the skull, neck, eye, sinuses
- Cranial Neuralgia
- Unclassifiable

Headaches Due to Disease vs. Headaches Due to Dysfunction

The first four categories are *"Primary Headache Disorders"*. In other words, they occur *"simply because"* (ultimately they are due to something but they are not due to another disease). Tests are usually normal, suggesting that they are not due to changes in the brain's structure, but rather due to changes in brain (or scalp, or vessel, etc.) function. The remainder, (aside from the last group), can be classified as **"Secondary Headaches"** or *headaches due to other diseases*.

It is with the last category that I will be dealing with this article.

Diseases can cause headaches in several ways. One way is by

causing increased pressure in the brain such as with a brain tumour or hydrocephalus (swelling of the fluid-filled cavities of the brain). Any time there is increased pressure, pulling (*"traction"*) of the pain sensitive blood vessels and nerve endings occurs, and pain therefore results. Another way pain develops is from inflammation or irritation of the meninges (or linings of the brain) as in meningitis or in a hemorrhage from an aneurism. Inflammation in the arteries of the scalp and other blood vessels can lead to headaches such as in conditions known as *"Temporal Arteritis"* or *"Vasculitis"*.

> *"headaches caused by tumours are said to be around 1%."*
>
> *Any headache problem is cause for concern and should be taken seriously and chronic headaches should be investigated with a headache neurologist or a physician.*

Headaches can also occur because of low cerebrospinal fluid pressure states in the brain such as for example following a lumbar puncture. In this instance, cerebrospinal fluid is removed through needle insertion between the bones of the spine. This removes some of the fluid that cushions the brain, causing the brain to sag. This leads to traction or pulling on the linings of the brain and to dilation (bulging) of the blood vessels. Headaches can also occur when nerves in the head and scalp are directly affected by inflammation, tumours, or other irritating factors (such as occurs in the various neuralgias). Headaches can also occur because of problems in the teeth, sinuses and scalp itself. Most people are surprised to hear that brain tissue itself is not pain sensitive. This is why a neurosurgeon can operate on someone's brain, while they are awake, without them feeling pain when only the outer layers of the skull and meninges have been anesthetized ("frozen").

How Does The Doctor Know What Type of Headache The Patient Has?

When a patient sees a physician they are often concerned about having an underlying disease such as a brain tumour. However, most headaches are the **primary type** and are **not** due to another disease. Taking a good history from the patient and performing a thorough physical examination is the best way to sort things out. This is why it is so important for you to come prepared to your appointment and to be able to give an accurate description of your symptoms.

One common myth is that the more severe a headache, the more likely it is to be due to a disease. Another is that the longer you have had a headache the more likely it is to be due to a disease. In fact, one could argue that the opposite is true. When your physician is trying to sort out whether your headache is due to disease or due to dysfunction, they will look at the factors which precipitate and relieve the pain and they will look for other features in your past medical history and family history that might give them clues. Certain "red flags" may lead your physician to be worried about a secondary cause as to the headache such as very abrupt onset of headache; headache pattern that changes; progressive headaches for no obvious reasons; headaches associated with protracted vomiting or with fever; new onset of headache in an elderly person; headaches precipitated by a "Valsalva Maneuver" (this is something that occurs when you sneeze, cough or strain); headaches triggered by changes in position, head turning or exercise; headaches that awaken one in the night; headaches associated with other neurologic signs or symptoms such as confusion or changes in your thinking; headaches associated with "systemic symptoms" (symptoms related to the body as a whole such as fever, weight loss, muscle aches).

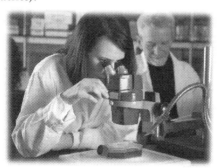

Of course, a benign headache, (like migraine), can be severe and may be associated with vomiting. It may come on in adult life, it may worsen with coughing, sneezing or straining, and it may be associated with other neurologic symptoms, etc. As you can see this leads to some of the difficulties associated with diagnosis. However, when patients describe a typical history of migraines and their examination is normal, it is very unlikely for them to have anything other than just migraines. In fact, an adept physician can detect headaches due to disease fairly accurately simply based on the history provided by the patient and physical examination. Sometimes investigations are warranted (when things don't fit a neat pattern, when "red flags" appear etc.) but most of the time this is to provide reassurance to the patient, family or doctor in cases where there are some features that raise concern.

Headaches that are associated with neurological symptoms can also be problematic. While migraine may be associated with many neurological and other, even systemic symptoms, including mental symptoms and confusion, so that while these symptoms may be associated with a serious disease, many of them might also be associated with migraine.

Listed below is a review of the different types of headaches due to disease.

A. Post-Traumatic and Headaches After Head Injuries

Headaches following whiplash injury or from degenerating discs in the neck fall into this category. The cause of these headaches is unclear and ultimately they are not a dangerous condition although they can lead to considerable disability. The headache can resemble migraine headaches or may have features of both migraine and tension-type headaches. Often the pain starts in the neck and may be accompanied by neck pain/or stiffness. The treatment must deal with the entire post-traumatic syndrome and can be quite challenging. Rarely is a headache (contrary to popular belief), due to a "pinched nerve in the neck".

Post-Traumatic symptoms can include dizziness, memory loss, concentration difficulties, sleep disturbances, depression, and personality changes, etc.

B. Headaches Associated With "Space Occupying Lesions":

By space occupying lesions we mean essentially tumours, cysts, abscesses, large blood clots and other masses which take up space in the brain and increase pressure in the brain. Although these headaches are very disconcerting, they are actually quite rare. Indeed most "space occupying lesions" can present with symptoms **other than** headaches such as nausea and/or vomiting, confusion, seizures, memory problems, personality changes, balance difficulties, weakness, numbness, and patients almost invariably show abnormalities on examination, such as "papilledema" (swelling of the optic nerves which can be seen when looking into the eye). However, **most** "Space Occupying Lesions" do have a headache.

The main feature that allows your doctor to tell that you are dealing with a "lesion", is that when it does produce a headache, it is the type that just keeps worsening; it usually does not wax and wane without treatment. Both a CT scan and an MRI can diagnose a space occupying lesion. Therefore, if someone has a headache with disserting features and one does an MRI scan, if the CT scan is negative and the examination is negative one can conclude that if this patient does have a brain tumour, then it is not the source of their headaches.

C. Headaches Due To Ear, Nose And Dental Disease

Headaches can occur because of sinusitis, both chronic and acute (long term & short term), a "septal contact syndrome" (a situation where the bone which runs down the middle of the nose makes contact with one of the side walls of the nose) or even because of nasal congestion from allergies. Most people are misled by the location of their head pain in the centre of the face or above an eye and by symptoms of nasal congestion into thinking they have something different, such as migraines. True "acute sinusitis" is actually rare (fortunately) and is usually accompanied by feelings of malaise, fever, and a yellow-green discharge. Another factor that complicates the issue is that migraines often respond to over-the-counter "sinus-medication".

Some difficulties can include concentration problems, sleep disturbances, depression and personality changes. The treatment must deal with the entire post-traumattic syndrome and can be quite challenging.

D. Headaches Due To Irritation Of The Meninges

The meninges are the lining around the brain. They are quite sensitive and anything that inflames, tugs on, or irritates the meninges can lead to a headache. These headaches tend to have a typical pattern with stiffening of the neck and often times spinal fluid tests reveal some abnormality. Some of the common causes of "meningeal headaches" are infections (bacterial, viral, and others), cancer, sarcoidosis (a rare inflammatory disease that can affect all organs of the body,) hemorrhage into the fluid space of the meninges (subarachnoid hemorrhage due to a ruptured aneurysm), chemical headaches from certain drugs, in particular some anti-inflammatories (surprisingly), and rare tumours that leak irritating substances into the cerebrospinal fluid space (the fluid that circulates in and around the brain).

E. Headaches of Cerebrovascular Origin

These are headaches caused by problems with the blood vessels. Blood vessel problems can lead to headaches in various ways. One such way is by causing bleeding around the brain or into the brain from an aneurysm or vascular malformation for instance.

Vasculitis or inflammation of the blood vessels of the brain can cause headaches as well as tearing of the blood vessels (what is known as "arterial dissection") and can lead to headaches. High blood pressure causes headaches only rarely and only when it is very high. Most of the time when patients have a headache and are noted to have high blood pressure **it is the headache that is causing the high blood pressure** (as any source of pain tends to cause the blood pressure to rise) rather than the opposite. Some patients who have strokes because of blocked blood vessels complain of headaches. Headache occurs on over 50% of ischemic and stroke-related illnesses. When they do we are not really certain why. It may be because blood flow is diverted to other vessels which dilate.

F. Medication Overuse Headache (One Very Important Cause of Headaches!)

This will be fully covered in Chapter 9 - Medication Overuse and therefore I will not go into it at this time.

Certain headaches occur more commonly in certain age groups. **In children** most headaches are still migraines but headaches can be associated with certain serious diseases such as brain tumours, meningitis, pseudotumour (a condition that mimics a brain tumour and leads to raised pressure in the brain but without the actual tumour). **In the elderly**, one needs to be concerned more about space occupying lesions (because these patients are at greater risk of tumours and of hemorrhages in the brain) and about stroke and high blood pressure. Elderly patients also tend to have more "systemic diseases" such as respiratory problems, anemia, blood sugar problems, and glaucoma that can lead to headaches. Degenerative disease of the neck is also quite common in the elderly. Finally, **temporal arteritis** (see Chapter 11 - People Over 50) is a condition that presents in patients over the age of 60 and is potentially dangerous because it can lead to visual loss and other neurological problems.

Other than the primary headaches there are over 300 causes of headache.

This review does not pretend to be comprehensive and cover all diseases. There are many diseases that have been left out. However, it is more important to realize that most headaches are not due to diseases, but are "idiopathic" or primary. A skilled physician is your best tool in ruling out headaches caused by disease.

Headaches Due to Disease was updated and reviewed by Dr. Joel Saper, Michigan Headache & Neurological Institute, Ann Arbor, Michigan

*Acute Medicines and Ergot Derivatives in this chapter have been reviewed by Irene Worthington, Drug Information Pharmacist, Headache Network Canada, Toronto, Canada with further reviews from Dr. Gary Shapero, The Shapero Markham Headache & Pain Treatment Centre, Unionville, Ontario, Canada

4

How a Headache is Treated by Preventative Medicines

Prevent the Next Attack in Frequency, Severity, & Length

What are preventative medicines?

Preventative medicines are medications that are taken daily, by some sufferers, to reduce the frequency, severity and length of the migraine attacks.

When the physician is contemplating starting preventative medication for migraine, the risks and benefits must be carefully reviewed with the patient. There are numerous choices among the types of medications that can be made, and through careful consultation, the physician and patient can reach a decision together.

As with taking any medication there are benefits, and side effects the patient should be aware of before deciding on medical treatment. These will subsequently be reviewed.

Why are Preventative Medicines used? What is their purpose?

Preventative Medicines, otherwise commonly referred to as Migraine Prophylaxis is often used in conjunction with acute medicines - see Chapter 3 - Acute Medicines, as a way of helping some sufferers better manage their headaches. The goals of prophylactic migraine therapy are to lesson headache frequency and severity, reduce the need for acute medication and reduce disability.

Migraine guidelines recommend initiating preventative medications when the number of attacks exceeds 3-4 per month. However, in the patient who only has 2 migraines per month with long duration of 4 days each, one may also consider prevention here.

Alternatively, if their acute abortive medications are not working well enough for them, or in situations or migraine specific therapy is contraindicated such as in pregnancy, or in heart disease, consideration to prevention could be given. Most preventative medicines were borrowed from other areas of medicine. Often, people have other afflictions and they might also be migraine sufferers. By chance, when taking the preventative medicine for something else, it has helped to reduce the frequency of a sufferer who gets migraine headaches.

Many of the migraine preventative medications are used for other conditions, such as epilepsy, hypertension or depression. With so many different medications to choose from it is sometimes difficult for the clinician to know which medication to choose for his/her patient. In some cases, one medication may be used to treat two existing conditions. For example in the patient with hypertension, the physician may choose a betablocker which is normally used to treat blood pressure but is also a very effective migraine prevention agent.

The choice of a preventative medication should depend on the headache types, the side effect profile, the potential drug interactions of other medications the patient is taking, comorbid conditions and patient and physician preferences.

These are some basic principles that must be observed in preventative treatment management. Treatment must be started at a low dose with gradual increase in the dose to a therapeutic level before it is abandoned and an adequate amount of time, ie. minimum six weeks allowed on the medication before it is deemed a failure. Finally if one medication fails one can always try another!

Although the medications listed below likely won't eliminate severe headaches; their goal is to make them less frequent and less intense and therefore, more manageable. Preventative medication is often combined with abortive medication, from the headache specialist. The goal of "prevention" is a 50% reduction in headache severity and frequency. Migraines can be controlled not cured. Patients should be given realistic expectations about treatment.

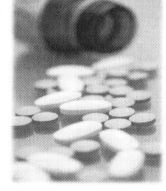

When your doctor chooses a preventative medicine for you he/she must consider - your age, sleeping patterns, other illnesses you may have, stomach absorption, and allergies, and your overall feelings about taking medicines.

Common misunderstandings when taking preventative medicines:

- always tell your doctor of any side-effects you may be experiencing

- give the medication a reasonable time frame to become effective by starting at a low dosage - making a gradual increase for at least 6 weeks.

- take the preventative medication even when you are "headache free".

- report any "non-pharmacological approaches" that you are taking, to your doctor, as this could influence the headache preventative prescribed

- don't just stop the medication because you may believe it is not working; always consult a physician first.

- never share your medication with other sufferers as each persons body is unique and responds differently to medicines.

Emotional distress that contributes to a headache, and its severity, is covered in Chapter 7 - Headache Triggers, Caffeine & Social Support. Nonpharmacological approaches can sometimes be very effective adjunctive treatments in achieving maximal headache manageability. (See Chapter 5 - Alternative Approaches and Botox)

Categories of Preventative Medicines

Categories are:
>Antidepressants
>Beta-Blockers
>Nonsteroidal Anti-inflammatories (NSAIDs)
>Calcium Channel Blockers
>Methysergide
>Monomine Oxidase Inhibitors (MOIs)
>Anticonvulsants.

Antidepressants

Among the most commonly prescribed preventative headache medications are the antidepressants. Their therapeutic value was discovered by chance for migraine sufferers in the 1970s. The single most common of the "antidepressant family of medicines" is amitriptyline (brand name, Elavil). Amitriptyline is a tricyclic antidepressant. There are other antidepressants used to aid migraine sufferers in finding headache relief, but Amitriptyline is the most utilized in the antidepressant family of medications.Its usefulness is that it helps to promote sleep and controlled anxiety. However, its limitation is drowsiness and weight gain.

Beta-Blockers

Officially called "Beta-andrenergic-Blockers", these medicines are widely used in migraine prevention. The Beta-Blocker most common to the general public is Propanolol (Inderal).

Clinical drug trials have shown that Propranolol is effective in the treatment of migraine prevention, for reducing frequency and severity of headache. It should <u>not</u> be given to patients with asthma as it may cause an exacerbation.

Beta-Blockers can also be useful to headache sufferers who additionally have high blood pressure, as well as migraines - as these medicines can help both ailments.

Nonsteroidal Anti-Inflammatory Drugs (NSAIDs)

Ibuprofen, Naproxen and Aspirin are a few examples of NSAID's.

If one NSAID does not work another is usually tried before jumping to another category of headache medicine. NSAIDS are generally well tolerated although they must be used with caution in patients with gastric reflux and should be avoided in patients with peptic ulcer disease.

Naproxen is sometimes given to headache sufferers to help diminish that "itch" from ingesting too much over-the-counter medicine, commonly associated with rebound headache or medication overuse headache. (See Chapter 9 - Chronic Daily Headache, Fibromyalgia and Chronic Fatigue Syndrome). Although NSAIDS may be very effective in migraine prevention for the short term, use in long term prophylaxis is not recommended.

Calcium Channel Blockers

Flunarizine (Sibelium) is the only Calcium Channel Blocker

that has been proven to be effective for migraine sufferers - in clinical trials. One side effect to watch out for may be depression and weight gain. Headache physicians also use Verapamil as a preventative for migraine, without great evidence for it in clinical trials.

Methysergide

Methysergide is thought to block the inflammatory and vessel-constricting effects of serotonin - the neurotransmitter significantly responsible for a migraine headache attack.

This medicine generally requires a four to six week drug hiatus or holiday **every** six months. Although rare, it has been associated with fibrosis, pulmonary, retroperitoneal, and for this use is not commonly prescribed. Good clinical evidence to support its benefit is minimal.

Monamine Oxidase Inhibitors (MAOs)

Monamine Oxidase Inhibitors are rarely used in the prevention of migraine. Many headache specialists do not use them on migraine patients as these specialists are concerned with dietary concerns causing severe side-effects. Evidence to support their use is also minimal.

Anticonvulsants or Antiseizure Medications

Examples of anticonvulsants would include Topamax (Topiramate), Valproic Acid (Depakote) and Gabapentin (Periactin). There is good evidence that suggests that all three of these medicines are effective for migraine prevention. There are good clinical trials for all three of the above anticonvulsants showing a good clinical response with reduction in frequency, and severity. Topiramate in doses of 100-200 milligrams is a very effective migraine prophylatic. The physician is advised to start at a low dose and titrate slowly over 1-2 months to a therapeautic level. Potential side effects may include numbness of digits, may be dose related and may settle down after a few weeks with loss of taste or weight loss. One of the more troublesome side effects may be cognitive which may affect short-term memory, word-finding and mood. Patients need to inform their families of these potential side-effects, as they may not be aware. These may settle down with time, in some cases circumstances. Rarely the medication needs to be discontinued.

Valproic Acid is also a very well known anticonvuisant with a long history in the epilepsy world. Its use in migraine prevention has also been supported by good clinical drug trials. Doses may vary from 750-1500 milligrams per day. The most troublesome side effects are weight gain, potential hair loss and possible gastric upset.

Gabapentin similarily has demonstrated good efficacy and good tolerability. Side-effects for this medication may be some drowsiness or weight gain.

Reviewed by Dr. Rose Giammarco, Hamilton Headache Clinic, Hamilton, Ontario, Canada

Botulinum Toxin Injection

Botox as a preventative treatment has been covered extensively at the end of Chapter 5 - see Chapter 5 - Alternatives and Botox. Also, there is a button called Botox on the Help for Headaches website at www.headache-help.org with an article from a neurologist with special interest in headache management, from McMaster University in Hamilton, Canada. The article can be printed off so it can be read later.

Alternative Preventatives

The alternatives that are used in migraine prevention are Feverfew Leaf, Vitamin B2 and Magnesium. (These are covered in Chapter 5 - Alternatives)

Multifactorial Approach

One migraine association in the US suggests:

"However, the best approach to Migraine management is what MAGNUM calls a MULTIFACTORAL approach, which involves addressing all four aspects of Migraine health care: preventive treatment, trigger management, abortive treatment, and general pain management."

The following article was reprinted with permission from "Headache Relief" by Dr. Fred Sheftell.

Drugs: Effects, Effectiveness, and Side Effects:

What's Wrong With Drugs --
And What's Right With Them

We always use great caution and care in prescribing medications for our patients. On the one hand, we know that medications may have side effects, and in rare cases may even make headaches worse. On the other hand, we know that medications may offer a patient the first relief from headache he or she has had for a long time. In some cases, medication may offer the breathing space to make other changes in headache patterns, or may offer a safety net to reassure a patient that there is a last-ditch defense against the pain. In other cases, especially for patients with chronic headache problems, medication is the cornerstone of our treatment.

Basically, medication has four major types of effect. It may elevate the pain threshold; that is, physical processes remain the same, but the person's experience of pain is blocked. It may modify muscle tone, causing tight muscles to relax or preventing them from contracting in certain ways. It may decrease inflammation of the brain, nerves and blood vessels, encouraging them to constrict or dilate. It can also increase the availability of certain neurotransmitters and stimulate certain nerves to react, counteracting the usual biochemical processes that produce headaches.

All of these effects may be accomplished to some extent by drug-free methods...(such as) biofeedback, psychological approaches and relaxation techniques, exercise and massage, and diet. In general, the "side-effects" of these techniques are overwhelmingly positive, while the side effects of most medication are at best only slightly annoying, though they can usually be dealt with by a change in dose or medication.

Headache Triggers

A terrific way to avoid migraines in the first place is to use "trigger-avoidance" and never set the migraine in place to begin with.

Below I have listed a very brief list of triggers (reprinted with permission from an International Headache Neurologist), Dr. Lawrence Robbins. I explain "migraine triggers" more thoroughly in Chapter 7 - Headache Triggers, Caffeine and Social Support.

Common Migraine Triggers

- Overwhelming "daily headache"
- Stress, worry, depression, and anger
- Some foods
- Weather and seasonal changes, such as humidity or high heat
- Smoke, perfume, gasoline, paint, organic solvents, and other strong odors

- Hunger
- Fatigue or lack of sleep
- Hormonal factors such as menstruation, birth control pills, pregnancy, menopause, estrogens
- Oversleeping and excessive sleep
- Bright lights, such as glaring artificial lights or bright sunlight
- Head Trauma
- Altitude
- Motion, experienced during car rides or amusement park rides, for example

Please note that identifying your headache trigger and using "trigger avoidance" is a very powerful way to prevent your next migraine. This is a short list of potential migraine triggers, and a much more comprehensive list can be found on Chapter 7 - Headache Triggers, Caffeine & Social Support.

The following article "Current Trends in Migraine Prophylaxis" was reprinted with permission from Dr. Lawrence Robbins, Robbins Headache Clinic, Northbrook, Illinois.

A variety of drugs from diverse pharmacological classes are in use for migraine prevention. Traditionally, they have been discovered by serendipity. Examples include ßß-adrenergic blockers, anticonvulsants, tricyclic antidepressants, and serotonin receptor antagonists. The mechanisms of action of migraine preventive drugs are multiple but it is postulated that they converge on two targets: (1) inhibition of cortical excitation; (2) restoring nociceptive dysmodulation. The antiepileptic drugs (e.g. topiramate, valproate, gabapentin), calcium channel blockers such as verapamil, and inhibitors of cortical spreading depression are some examples of drugs that reduce neuronal hyperexcitability. On the other hands, modulators of the serotonergic and adrenergic systems and cholinergic enhancing drugs may restore descending nociceptive inhibition and play a role in migraine prevention. To date, Level 1 evidence and clinical experience favor the use of the antidepressant amitriptyline, and anticonvulsants divalproex and topiramate, and the ßß-adrenergic blockers Propranolol, Timolol and Metoprolol as first line migraine preventive drugs. The evidence for others (e.g., verapamil) is not as strong. Migraine preventive drugs have varying degrees of adverse effects, some of which could be limiting, and their efficacy should be balanced with their risks of adverse effects, patients expectations and desires, and compliance. It is hoped that future migraine preventive drugs target migraine mechanisms more specifically, which could well enhance the therapeutic index.

Dr. Lawrence Robbins furthers writes in his book - Headache Help: A complete guide to understanding headaches and the medicines that relieve them. Reprinted with permission from pages 262-63

- You might become frustrated by the lack of effectiveness or by the side effects of daily preventatives. Remember: 50 percent (at most) of patients achieve long-term relief with preventatives. Knowing this should allow you to realize that if they don't help, it's not your fault.

- If you have chronic headaches, understand that the "cure" may not be total. You may still have headaches everyday, but they may become less severe. Ask yourself if you have gone from severe to moderate (from a 10 down to a 7) or from a moderate to mild (from a 7 to a 4). If you show improvement, all the medication should not be changed.

- Remember, good headache therapy, just like other challenges, requires patience, persistence, perseverance.

- Learn how to cope with stress effectively, whether through cognitive strategies that can be learned from self-help books or in using relaxation or breathing techniques, exercise, yoga, massage, footbaths, or whatever works for you. Don't overload yourself with too many obligations. Learn to say no.

5

Alternative Treatments including Migralex and Botox Treatments

Are alternatives safe and reliable?

Migralex
by Alexander Mauskop, MD, FAAN
New York Headache Center
30 East 76 Street
New York, NY 10021
Tel: 212.794.3550
www.nyheadache.com

Migralex - A new generation of headache relief - find it at
www.migralex.com

Migralex is a new over-the-counter headache medication which offers several advantages over older medications. It combines two safe and proven therapies in a unique formulation which delivers excellent relief with few side-effects.

About 30 million Americans suffer from migraine headaches and many more have tension-type, sinus and hangover headaches. Over-the-counter medications provide relief to some of these sufferers, but for many they fall short. Prescription drugs are very expensive, carry a higher risk of side effects and also work for only 60% of patients.

None of the prescription or over-the-counter drugs addresses a major underlying cause of headaches, which is magnesium deficiency. Research indicates that up to half of migraine sufferers have magnesium deficiency. Stress is a common trigger for headaches and stress has been shown to deplete magnesium. Alcohol is another powerful depleter of magnesium and hangover headaches are thought to be triggered by this effect. Irritable bowel syndrome, asthma, diabetes and many other chronic medical problems result in loss of magnesium. Magnesium deficiency contributes to PMS symptoms, muscle cramps, coldness of extremities and many other symptoms. Acute strokes are being treated with magnesium infusions. Many brain cell functions are dependent on the presence of magnesium.

Migraine and other types of headaches are accompanied by inflammatory changes in the brain. Aspirin has been proven to relieve even severe migraines in several large studies. It is the only anti-inflammatory drug that does not cause heart attacks. In fact it prevents heart attacks and strokes and may have many other benefits, including prevention of Alzheimer's disease, colon and other cancers.

Using only an anti-inflammatory pain killer, acetaminophen or a prescription migraine drug does not address the complex sequence of events, which occur in the brain of a headache sufferer and provides only modest relief. Migralex combines magnesium, which corrects the deficiency and improves function of brain cells and a century-old anti-inflammatory drug, aspirin in a unique and rapidly acting headache medication.

ALTERNATIVE TREATMENTS FOR HEADACHES
reprinted with permission from healthology. com

The successful treatment of conditions ranging from the common cold to many cancers remains beyond the reach of modern medicine, despite its tremendous advances. It is not surprising, then, that patients seek a variety of alternative or complimentary therapies. Complementary techniques are those that lack definitive proof of efficacy and are not accepted by the medical mainstream. While many treatments widely used in modern medicine also lack scientific proof, they are not considered complementary or alternative because of their wide acceptance by the medical establishment.

Headaches & Alternatives

While the experience of an occasional headache may be universal and usually is tolerable, chronic headache is an important cause of distress and disability. The vast majority of people who suffer from headaches have either tension-type or migraine headaches. Headache only recently began to receive attention from the pharmaceutical industry and organized medicine. Selective migraine medicines have revolutionized treatment of migraine and dramatically changed the lives of millions of people. But some have begun to explore complementary methods. . .as an alternative. Most headache sufferers, however, have never seen a physician and may turn to complementary treatments, which seem cheaper, safer, (though this may not always be the case), and more holistic. Non-invasive does not mean without side-effects.

In numerous double-blind treatment trials, a large proportion (30-40%) of headache sufferers respond favorably to placebo. This "placebo effect" can account for completely useless therapies being effective in some sufferers. If a particular therapy appears to be clearly ineffective, but at the same time is harmless and inexpensive, I would not discourage an interested sufferer from trying such an approach, in hopes of a favorable placebo response.

Types of complementary placebo response.

Acupuncture

This ancient method has recently received a boost in popularity because of the consensus statement by a panel convened by the

National Institutes of Health. This statement strongly suggests that acupuncture is a legitimate therapy proven to be effective for some conditions and deserving additional studies for others. The panel concluded that nausea and acute dental pain clearly respond to acupuncture, while many painful conditions, including headaches, may respond to acupuncture but require additional studies.

Acupuncture treatment is done using very thin disposable needles, which cause very little discomfort or pain. In sufferers with chronic headaches treatment involves ten or more weekly 20-minute sessions. Electrical stimulation of the needles is frequently used instead of the traditional twirling of the needles.

Double-blind study of acupuncture is very difficult because blinding for insertion of a needle is impossible, and inserting the needles into non-acupuncture points has been shown to relieve pain.

Despite the lack of definitive proof of its efficacy, acupuncture has a significant potential to help some patients with headaches. Issues of cost, convenience and patient preferences should be taken into account when deciding on this treatment.

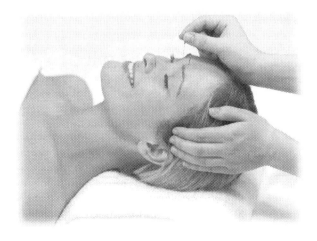

Mind-Body Techniques

Biofeedback is another therapy where definitive proof will be hard to obtain. Most specialty headache clinics offer biofeedback, which strongly suggests that a large number of sufferers benefit from it (but does not prove its efficacy).

Biofeedback is only one of many relaxation and stress management techniques which can be equally effective if strictly adhered to. This is a big "if". Biofeedback is a preferred technique because it gives the sufferer a structure and a therapist, who acts as a coach.

The essence of biofeedback, which is often combined with behavioural modification, is to teach a sufferer how to encounter stress without adverse physiological effects. A typical course of biofeedback consists of 8-10 weekly 30-45 minute sessions. Learning to control body functions such as temperature can be achieved only by first learning to relax the skeletal muscles. This is achieved through progressive relaxation, visualization and breathing techniques. The practice sessions can only be a few seconds or minutes long, and have to be very frequent. A conscious effort is required in the first few weeks of training, but gradually self-monitoring and very brief relaxation techniques become a subconscious habit. This appears to allow many sufferers to lower tension throughout the day and this results in fewer headaches. Children are especially adept at biofeedback. They can learn not only how to prevent their headaches in 4 to 5 sessions, but at times can learn how to stop their headache once it begins.

Nutritional Therapies

Dietary approaches to the treatment of migraines are widely advocated, but have very little scientific basis, which places them in the category of complementary methods. Dietary avoidance is a widely advocated strategy. Migraine can be triggered in susceptible individuals by tyramine-containing foods, some food additives and sugar substitutes, as well as by skipping meals. Some sufferers report their headaches get better with elimination of wheat, sugar, or milk products from their diets. While we do not have scientific proof, it is possible to speculate on why these dietary changes may work. If the sufferer is so inclined there is no reason to discourage him/her from trying these dietary changes, which are usually safe and inexpensive. Strict vegetarian and other usual diets, on the other hand, can lead to vitamin B12 and other deficiencies, which can make headaches worse and cause other health problems.

Magnesium is a vital element which plays an important role in the pathogenesis of migraines. Many studies have found low magnesium levels in the serum and tissues of migraine sufferers. In one study, an intravenous infusion of 1 gram of magnesium sulfate was given to 40 consecutive sufferers with acute migraine. Twenty-one (53%) had good and sustained relief of their headache. Of the responders, 86% had low serum ionized magnesium levels, while of the non-responders only 16% had low values. A study of intravenous magnesium in the treatment of cluster headaches suggests a possible 40% success rate in this difficult-to-treat disorder. Oral magnesium supplementation was attempted as preventative therapy of migraines in three double-blind trials. Two of the three trials were positive, while one was negative. The negative study might have used a more poorly absorbed salt of magnesium. The absorption of various salts of magnesium has not been studied, so it is difficult to recommend a specific product to patients interested in trying magnesium for their headaches. Magnesium oxide, magnesium diglycinate and slow-release magnesium chloride seems to work for some sufferers when used. Consult a doctor.

Wider availability of serum ionized magnesium testing may enable us to identify patients who have low ionized magnesium levels and who are most likely to benefit from magnesium supplementation. In order to remove magnesium from the list of complementary therapies and move it into the mainstream we need large trials of unequivocally proving its efficacy.

Riboflavin or vitamin B2 has been reported to relieve migraine headaches better than placebo. The maximum effect was achieved after three months of daily intake of riboflavin. The study involved only 55 sufferers, but the treatment is very benign and potentially very effective, which makes riboflavin a good candidate for further extensive trials.

Herbal Remedies

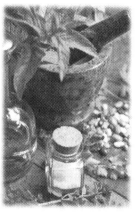

Feverfew is the only herbal remedy studied in double-blind fashion. In a trial of 24 patients, a daily dose of feverfew was found to be better than placebo as a preventative therapy for migraines, though the difference was not dramatic. Because feverfew is fairly safe and may help some sufferers, this is the herb to recommend to sufferers interested in herbal medicines. Migra-Lieve is a product made by National Science Corporation of America which contains magnesium, riboflavin and feverfew in one tablet. Having these three ingredients in one tablet greatly improves compliance and has been effective for many of my patients. However, my involvement started only after I became convinced that it helps my patients.

Guarana is a relatively recent import from Brazil, which is being used for headache relief. It may very well have some analgesic properties because of its high caffeine content. See Chapter 7 - Caffeine. However, daily caffeine consumption is one of the leading causes of Medication Overuse Headaches. See Chapter 9 – Chronic Daily Headache - Medication Overuse. Guarana and other caffeine-containing foods, drinks and medications should be avoided in patients with frequent headaches.

Anecdotal reports suggest the ingestion of ginger, gingko or valerian root, all of which are well tolerated, may help some sufferers with headaches.

Aromatherapy

Aromatherapy may not appear far-fetched if we consider how much of our brain is devoted to olfaction (smelling) and how strong odors can almost instantly induce a migraine.

A double-blind study of healthy volunteers showed that an external application of peppermint extract raises pain threshold and has strong relaxing effects, while eucalyptus has calming and relaxing effects and improves cognitive performance without analgesic effect. Another study which used peppermint oil for tension headaches showed positive results. This gives some scientific support to a variety of topical products being promoted for the treatment of headaches.

Homeopathy

Homeopathy is based on an unproved concept of using extremely small amounts of substances (usually herbal), which in large amounts can induce the symptoms that are being treated. Since the treatment is extremely benign and relatively inexpensive it can be tried by sufferers who believe it might help them.

Physical Approaches

Regular and frequent aerobic exercise as a treatment for headaches is impossible to study in a double-blind trial and would require a very large comparative trial to confirm efficacy. However, there is little doubt that it offers effective relief for many stress-provoked conditions including headaches. Other unproven but anecdotally effective modalities include the application of heat and cold, massage and many other similar techniques. As long as they are safe and affordable, sufferers should not be discouraged from trying them.

Chiropractic manipulation has several potential benefits, which must be weighed against possible complications. Controlled studies in tension headaches have yielded mixed results, while small trials looking at migraine prevention have been encouraging. A person's feelings about the treatment need to be considered as well as sufferer compliance. Always consult with a physician before commencing any treatment whether prescription, alternative, over-the-counter.

Non-Pharmacological Approaches to Migraine (sections)
by Judith Anne Abdalla, M.D. F.R.C.P.(C)
Neurology
London, Canada

Hypnotherapy

Hypnotherapy (or self-hypnosis) is now becoming more common. It is not effective for everyone, and some time is required to learn to become hypnotized or to hypnotize oneself. Again, one of the difficulties is finding someone who is trained to do this. Hypnosis always involves imagery, visualization, goal-directed relaxation, self-suggestion, etc. The aim is to induce a trance-like state with a goal of focusing the trance or attention on a specific result such as relaxation, pain control, etc. Again, children seem to be better at entering a hypnotic state than many adults, but practice is an important feature.

Massage

Massage can be carried out in many different ways. One method is to simply massage or apply pressure with one's fingers to the painful area. Specifically trained registered massage therapists offer the best of improvement though. Aside from being quite a pleasant experience, the therapy can lead to a general sense of well-being and release of endorphins which can then relieve painful sensations. Once again, the cost is a limiting factor. Some private health insurance plans that are provincial, will absorb part of the cost of massage treatment if prescribed by a physician.

Trager™ is a gentler technique which may be more appropriate for those with muscle tenderness. Although it often leads to sense of general well-being and overall relaxation. Trager participants make no claims as to its efficacy in the treatment of migraine.

Naturopathy

Naturopathy is a treatment philosophy where a practitioner will combine various alternative techniques, including some techniques mentioned earlier plus dietary counseling, hydrotherapy, etc., to treat a particular ailment. The treatment plans are not scientifically based, are generally quite costly, are not covered by most insurance plans, and in some cases, may even be harmful.

In summary of all alternative approaches, one has to be just as careful one would when using a drug.

Proponents of alternative therapies may present glowing claims and often times traditional medical practitioners seem much more blunt, cold, and unduly critical of "alternative" practices.

Many approaches are valid while others are no better than placebo, while still others can actually harm you. I think it is important to have an open-minded physician and to develop a good relationship with him or her so that they may guide you amongst these various therapies and suggest one that might be helpful for you and your headache pattern.

Editor's note: it is important for the treating physician to

consider the sufferer's feelings toward an alternative approach, before beginning a treatment plan.

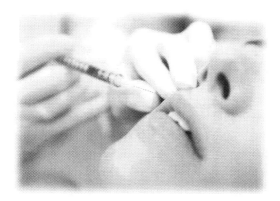

Botox Treatment

BOTOX FOR HEADACHE
by Dr. Rose Giammarco
Neurologist interested in Headache
McMaster University
Director of the Hamilton Headache Clinic
Hamilton, ON, Canada

Botulinum toxin is a neurotoxin produced by clostridium botulinum, the bacteria that thrive in poorly sterilized canned food and produces the severe food poisoning called botulism. This is the toxin that paralyzes nerves by blocking the release of a substance called acetylcholine - which blocks the muscles and prevents them from contracting thereby causing paralysis. The substance which is ingested in spoiled food and causes the illness is known as botulism.

However, in therapeutic uses, Botox is injected directly into the muscle rather than absorbed into the bloodstream. The dose is a fraction of that which causes botulism.

Botox is well known for its use in treatment of wrinkles. It has approval for use in treating facial tics and spasms, dystonia and other forms of spasticity in cerebral palsy for example. Its tolerability and safety record for these uses are excellent. The principle behind its use in this case is to relax tense or spastic muscles by blocking acetylcholine release which stimulates muscle contraction.

> **"the discovery of Botox for treatment of migraine was quite by accident"**

The discovery of Botox for treatment of migraine was quite by accident. Several patients who were using Botox for injection of wrinkles also happened to have migraine. They reported improvement in their headaches following injection of Botox to their brow and forehead muscles.

The mechanism of action is not entirely clear. One possibility is that Botox may decrease muscle contraction that may act as a trigger to migraine. Another theory is that Botox may act on a brain-related chemical-like substance P which is involved in pain and migraine mechanisms.

Careful trials studying migraine and chronic headache patients continue to examine the efficacy of Botox. Several small trials have been completed and results of a large placebo controlled trial are pending. The average dose is 100-200 units. The onset of action is usually within the first 2-3 weeks of injection. However, patients may require a set of 2-3 injections before maximum benefit is seen. Injections are spaced at 12 week intervals.

Safety is always a concern. However, Botox' record since 1989 is excellent. There is no systemic absorption as there is with oral medication; therefore no systemic side-effects are seen. Drooping eyelids can occur with improper injection technique but are transient.

Botox can be considered in patients when other migraine

treatments fail or are contraindicated. Cost depends on the number of units required. Safety and tolerability are excellent. Studies are ongoing to prove efficacy.

Note: Although Botox is technically a preventative medicine many sufferers think of it as an alternative so it was placed in this chapter.

6

Self-Help Strategies, Home Remedies, Workplace Issues & Meditation

It's 9pm and I'm home - how can I help myself?

Self-Help Strategies

Self-Help strategies can help you to cope with your headaches and they also have the extra added benefit of being free. However, they will "probably" only have minimal effect, but the focus is on lowering the pain threshold or preventing another headache or migraine attack from beginning.

Headaches are elusive....and are therefore difficult to treat and we all know how difficult they are to live with.

Further on in this chapter I will address a few suggestions for home remedies but first wanted to discuss "Red Flags".

Occasionally, headache symptoms are a concern and should be taken very seriously. Physicians call them "Red Flag Warnings" and they are:

- Your headaches begin abruptly with no history or reason (eg. fall)

- Your headaches are associated with dizziness, fatigue, vertigo

- Your headaches cause confusion or loss of consciousness

- You experience changes in vision

- Your headache is classified as "the worst ever"

- Your memory is altered and you become confused

- You have a fever associated with your headache (caution: headache is one of the associated features with fever)

- There is a sudden or drastic change in your "headache pattern"

This is probably the point where I interject and say how awfully important it is to you to learn your symptoms. Let's take the guesswork out of treating headaches.

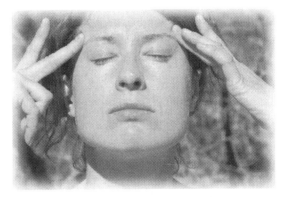

Some self-help strategies also might include:

- Join a support group for migraine or headache sufferers

- Research on the internet about free information, and locate a neurologist with a specialty in headache

- Purchase a book on headaches that you can "accidentally" leave on your coffee table for browsing through

- Go on the World Headache Alliance chat room discussion. World Headache Alliance - www.w-h-a.org

- Go to www.headache-help.org/headachelinks.html and search your suspected or diagnosed headache type, with the many headache websites that are linked

Caution should be used to not self-diagnose your condition. Remember that each sufferer is unique to their headache and an exact match may not be possible. Please be patient and understanding to both yourself and to your physician.

Changing your lifestyle can be difficult as routines, or patterns, are hard to break. Another factor is that often numerous people are involved so a solution is often difficult to arrange. Often changing your lifestyle can be costly, and requires additional effort, which is often hard to find.

A terrific self-help strategy is to practice exercise or aerobic respiration. A fit individual is in a better position to cope with a bad headache.

The following article on "Headache and Fitness" talks about the benefits of using mild-to-moderate exercise.

Headache and Fitness
by Brent Lucas
Help for Headaches
London, Canada

Regular exercise can greatly reduce your risk of headaches, and lack of regular exercise can leave you more susceptible to chronic headaches. Not only is exercise good at giving the headache sufferer an overall sense of well-being, it helps to promote good health. Exercise - depending on the individual - ranges from walking, treadmill, stationary bikes to aerobics. We now know that aerobic respiration increases our endorphins (our bodies' natural pain preventing chemicals) thereby reducing the sensation of pain felt.

Listed below are some major points for you to consider when making the critical decision to begin exercising. First, do it moderately and not severely. Moderation will always be a way to "ease" into your routine. It will also help you to maintain good headache prevention. Walking is also a terrific exercise and it brings with it the added benefit of social support when practiced with a friend. Second, use stretching exercises to warm up and maintain great flexibility so injury is less likely to happen. Always follow an instructor's advice on how far to stretch. Thirdly, slow down or stop if you experience any unusual discomfort or pain from exercising. Be sure to consult with an exercise specialist. He or she can suggest exercises that will not bring on pain. Fourth, always start an exercise routine consulting with a physician - then go under the supervision of a trained fitness professional.

Exercising can greatly reduce the frequency of headache attacks, and can increase your self-concept. The benefit here is not to just get in shape, or stay in shape, but to feel better all over - including your head! Take exercise seriously, and your headache pain will surely diminish - but the first step comes from you the sufferer.

Another very important self-help strategy is to "accept" that you have an ailment that is life-limiting and can flare up at times. It is important to be prepared for your next attack.

A good rule of thumb is to always be prepared - and often you will never have to rely on your back-up plans. On the other hand, when you go into a situation with no "alternate or back-up strategy" you may find yourself in jeopardy.

Exercise as a Migraine Trigger

Unfortunately, for a few migraine sufferers, exercise can actually induce a migraine. Exercise can sometimes lead to a headache when:

- You begin exercising abruptly and suddenly, thereby taking oxygen away from your body

- You forgot to drink plenty of water beforehand and dehydrate your body

- You have not eaten properly before the workout and therefore have low blood sugars

- You speed workout too quickly and hard, and your aching muscles can sometimes act as a headache trigger

There is no need to panic here as the pluses of exercise clearly outway the negatives.

Home Remedies

Has anyone shown you how to do deep breathing exercises? Their effects on reducing pain have long since been documented within the scientific community.

Here are a few suggestions for when it is 9pm and you are home:

- Drink a cup of coffee with caffeine (as long as your trigger is not caffeine)
  see Chapter 7 - caffeine (Caution: caffeine can be good news or bad news to your headache pattern)

- Practice exercises such as yoga that require deep breathing

- Practice imagery (there are free books in your library on imagery)

- Take OTC's such as tylenol or ibuprofen or acetaminophen as recommended on the bottle. (note: use caution to avoid medication overuse - see chapter 9)

- Put a cold compress on your head or neck

- Use a hot compress

- Try to lay flat and avoid bending over or doing any exertional activity

- Seek out a quiet, dark room

The obvious advantage of a home remedy is that they can be tried late at night, or on weekends or holidays, when a physician's office is closed. Another advantage is that they are usually free and are relatively easy to incorporate into your life.

Music is also a great way to learn to relax at home. There are a number of relaxational tapes available at most books stores to purchase. On the other hand, you might want to make your own tape to relax to. There are free music tapes to borrow from your local public library.

Warm baths or hot tubs can be a terrific way for the body to relax, especially when they are coupled with deep breathing exercises.

Another home remedy is to have your spouse or a friend, give you a massage. Remember to practice your breathing exercises at the same time.

Family support can really make a difference as to how the headache sufferer copes at home. Rather than isolating and blaming the sufferer, family support can bring with it a "we are going to get through this together" attitude.

Even if your family support is not real strong or understanding, there are a number of ways that you can help yourself, as I mentioned earlier.

It is very important to mention again, how beneficial "social support" is in maintaining good "headache control". Please see Chapter 7 - Social Support as that form of support can be a terrific home remedy as sometimes half the battle is just having someone "completely understand" what it is that you are going through.

Reducing stress is paramount to maintaining good headache control, and I have included an entire article from a physician in Chapter 12 on Stress.

Workplace Issues

Headaches in the Workplace

There are many factors as to why someone gets headaches in the workplace and it appears to be a very uneasy topic, especially for employers. And when you think about it - targeting problem areas not only assures effective quality control which is good for the employer and their company, but increases productivity and keeps the headache sufferer making all kinds of money. Yet it is a topic not well understood and it seems to be hardly ever raised at quality control meetings, until a crisis or very obvious crisis develops. But why?

Did you know that migraines are the #1reason why people miss time from work? According to Robbins, 2000 - 90% of headache sufferers can get help from a physician and 70% never bother to consult a physician.

Lost productivity in Canada remains at over 500 million lost annually (World Headache Alliance, 2007) and in the U.S. around $150 million per year (Sheftell, 2001) is lost due to worker absenteeism due to headache.

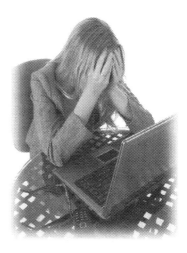

A typical headache sufferer can develop headaches from toxins or fumes present. Many headache researchers believe that these "odors" act as a powerful trigger to those that are migraine-prone. Much of the problem no longer exists, thank heavens due to health and safety regulations.

Bright fluorescent lights have long been documented as a trigger to set a migraine in process. Positioning a person in a not so highly lit area can benefit both the headache sufferer and the employer.

Certain positioning may bring relief from the stresses that contribute to back and neck pain. There are all kinds of ergonomic cushions, pillows, footrests available if your job requires you to sit for lengthy hours of time. Take a short walk whenever you can, as it will increase your blood circulation.

In our modern world, many use a computer. It is a much needed tool for the operation of companies. Travel-agents spend hours researching flight times - not to mention that constant staring at a computer screen can strain the eyeball.

When you stop and think about it, we spend as much time or sometimes even more time at work, than we do with our families. So doesn't it make sense to feel comfortable at your desk? Elimination of many headache types can be identified by reviewing your workplace for potential causes or triggers and that can be a good thing.

The employers fear can be spending money on ergonomics or special lighting. They are also cautious as to not wanting to bring this up for fear the sufferer starts "phoning in sick"... and since there is no real way to tell, employers are fearful for a good reason. But sufferers all agree that it is a problem and it deserves far more discussion. Most of us want to work, and desperately need the money. A call that "I have a headache" would impact on that very much. So I personally reject the phoning in sick fear - on behalf of the employer. The cost of repositioning furniture away from direct lighting can far outweigh the cost of lost productivity.

People who are afflicted with this awful illness which springs like a Tiger with usually little, or no warning - have no idea what kind of anxiety it can produce. It makes you feel crumby and to add insult to injury, is very misunderstood and not very recognized in the workplace.

A simple analogy is when a person gets something in the eye... or a hangnail....or a pulled muscle....they certainly complain a lot (and in most cases constantly). These are all discomforts that most of us feel from time to time. Why does a headache or migraine sufferer get scoffed at, and is sometimes called a malingerer?

What the public and in particular, employers, need to know is that in a migraine there is usually a certain set of chemical reactions that produce neurological symptoms. Certain foods, bright lights, hormones, environmental stimuli, etc. can all trigger a migraine but the cause is biochemical. And don't forget that illness is largely hereditary too. In defense of the sufferer... we did not ask for these afflictions, nor usually have any warning as to when they will strike.

A 3 year study in the UK found 13% of headache sufferers were unable to obtain or keep full-time work because of their pain condition (Stang et al, J Gen Intern Med 1998)
So what can I do to help myself and minimize upsetting my employer?

Joining a Health and Safety committee is a good start. Do your homework - from an employer's view point there is nothing worse than hearing some concerns and having nothing to back it up. Surfing the web can bring you lots of helpful information if you were ever to bring headaches in the workplace to your Health & Safety representative. You might try... workplace - headaches - Ontario - as a start. Move the keywords around. Try different keywords like "Absenteeism"! But put yourself in his or her shoes. Chances are they are not a sufferer and are like most of us... have their own slant on things. The odds of getting resistance are quite high and you may want to brace yourself for that.

Invite a guest speaker to come in and do a presentation. A ten minute video on headaches and worker absenteeism can speak volumes to your people and likely your boss. At that time, open it up to questions from the floor. This can be a great way to address an awkward topic, and not to feel so alone and intimidated.

For some unfortunates, headache rules their lives. Jobs are lost and that is the reality we all must live with. If that is your category see Chapter 13, Person's with a Disability.

Your job is sacred and it pays your bills, feeds your family and most likely has potential for advancement which means more money, and which generally means more comfort. Some companies will even pay for business trips. Advancement, unfortunately, usually means more headaches - no pun intended!

Approach this topic carefully and always "bring it up" casually, usually starting off with a positive stroke.

Remember, for some it can mean hearing about a potential problem for the first time. It's like you trying to understand a rare condition - be patient but also persistent. Now get to work!

Using Meditation to Manage Pain and Painful Emotions

by Barbaranne Branca, Ph.D., DABFE, DABFM
Michigan Headache and Neurological Institute
Ann Arbor, Michigan

With chronic pain, despair and guilt haunt many patients. A pain attack can persist for hours, days, even weeks. Pursuits with others--simple conversations, business dinners, games with children, or pursuits alone--doing a craft, enjoying the starry night sky—all activities are affected. Even if you stoically pursue life's activities, pain halves the pleasure and your spontaneous participation. You become depressed and frustrated and find yourself taking it out on others. You hear yourself responding with irritation to your spouse's question, with anger to your children's normal rushing through the house, and with anxiety as you make an excuse to withdraw from another family get-together. At work, the report is not as thorough as you know you are capable; in the afternoon, when the headache is worse, you function even less well, shuffling papers, putting off more complex tasks. You wrestle with yourself: do you take your medicine and risk being drowsy and even less effective? The inability to escape the pain once again, to avoid the headache disorder diagnosis altogether, and the far-reaching effect it has on your life, your work, and your loved ones causes tremendous suffering.

The myriad of decisions involved in managing a pain disorder on a day-to-day basis may seem overwhelming. Do I have enough energy to clean the closet without increasing my headache? Should I take an extra pain pill? How do I explain this to my son? Should I try to finish my taxes tonight? Conversely, it may seem that the pain takes away freedom to make decisions.

What do we do when we come to realize that there really is no "magic pill" for pain? Research and clinical experience shows that behavioral medicine can have a powerful effect on pain. Behavioral medicine examines and trains us to become aware of and to use the power of our minds and emotions on our physical health. One potent tool in recovering health is training in meditation.

Meditation is a form of paying attention, of becoming aware, and of directing consciousness. Dr. Kabat-Zinn directs the Stress Reduction Clinic at the University of Massachusetts Medical Center and uses mindfulness meditation to help patients who have chronic pain and stress. Mindfulness meditation is paying attention from moment-to-moment. This is carried out in conjunction with medical treatment to manage pain. Recommendations in this paper reinforce what has been shown in research — that the combination of both medical and behavioral medicine treatment is the most effective in pain management.

Dr. Kabat-Zinn's results speak for themselves. He has run 8 week training sessions in mindfulness meditation for many years. To examine the effect of mindfulness to modulate pain, a pain questionnaire (McGill-Melzack Pain Rating Index or PRI) is given. In one study, 72% of chronic pain patients reported a 33% reduction on their PRI scores. Scores on negative body image (how patients rated different parts of their body as problematic) were 30% lower by the end of the program. For people who have strong negative feelings about their body and are upset because their painful body/head holds them back from living, this is an impressive score in such a short period of time. A 30% improvement in the ability to engage in normal activities of daily living like cooking, driving, sex, and sleeping was reported. Mood was significantly improved (55%); negative feelings (anxiety, depression, anger) dropped, positive feelings increased, and preoccupation with health thoughts decreased. By the end of the program, people reported taking less pain medication, being more active, and feeling better overall.

Mindfulness meditation has a positive effect on multiple levels of a person's life. A large study (Reibel and colleagues, 2001) involved 136 patients, with a mix of chronic health problems. They learned mindfulness based stress reduction in an 8 week program and practiced meditation 20 minutes a day. Their responses were compared before and after on a health survey, medical symptom checklist, and psychological inventory. Health-related quality of life improved greatly; people reported increased energy, reduced body pain, less limited

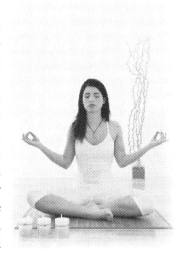

functioning, and increased ability to socialize. Medical symptoms were reduced 28%. Psychological relief was striking, with overall 38% reduction in distress, 44% reduction in anxiety and 34% reduction in depression. Follow-up with these patients a year later indicated that they had sustained these improvements.

A well-controlled study included 90 cancer patients (Speca and colleagues, 2000) who participated in mindfulness meditation to reduce stress and help with emotional distress. The patients had significantly reduced scores (65% less) on overall emotional distress--specifically depression, anxiety, anger, and confusion--and improved scores on vigor, when compared to the cancer patients in the control group (cancer patients who had not learned meditation). On a stress inventory, they reported 31% less stress than the controls. They had fewer cardiopulmonary and gastrointestinal symptoms.

On-the-job stress contributes to absenteeism, reduced productivity, injury, and affects pre-existing chronic disease. Stress management programs implemented at the work site that include relaxation and meditation, exercise, and biofeedback may reduce physiological symptoms, "for example, hypertension", increase job performance, and self-report of job satisfaction (Stein, 2001).

A pilot study (Creamer and colleagues, 2000) examined the effect of an eight-session treatment package with relaxation/meditation training and a Chinese movement therapy. Twenty fibromyalgia patients who completed 5 out of 8 of the cognitive-behavioral, educationally-based sessions improved as seen in pain threshold, tender points, and their responses on the Fibromyalgia Impact Questionnaire. This improvement continued when re-evaluated 4 months later.

There are many resources for learning mindfulness meditation stress reduction. Speak to your behavioral medicine psychologist about learning biofeedback, and relaxation. Supplement your discussion by reading Dr. Kabat-Zinn's book and other resources.

It is advisable to work with guidance. However, you can begin to create your own meditation practice.

1. Find a quiet, clean space. You are going to be sitting, either in a chair or on the floor. You have to be able to support your spine or make sure your spine is supported. Postural alignment is important and should convey dignity and calm. It is nice to beautify your space——put flowers on a table, for instance. Turn off the phone.

2. Practice for 10 minutes to start. Set an alarm so you do not have to worry about how much time has passed.

3. Focus on the breath. Feel your breath coming in and feel it going out. When your mind wanders, bring your attention back to your breath. You may find that your mind wanders 100 times in 10 minutes; just gently bring your attention back to your breath.

There are many techniques for mindfulness meditation and breathing, some of which are listed below. It really is possible for you to change how you respond to pain and to make a difference in managing your health.

1. Creamer, P; Singh, BB; Hochberg, MC; Berman, BM. Sustained improvement produced by nonpharmacologic intervention in fibromyalgia: results of a pilot study. Arthritis Care Res. 2000 Aug; 13(4):198-204.

2. Durgananda, S. The Heart of Meditation. South Fallsburg, NY:SYDA Foundation, 2002.

3. Kabat-Zinn, J. Full Catastrophe Living: Using the Wisdom and Your Body and Mind to Face Stress, Pain, and Illness. New York: Bantam, 1990.

4. Reibel, DK; Greeson, JM; Brainard GC; Rosenzweig S. Mindfulness-based stress reduction and health-related quality of

life in a heterogeneous patient population. Gen Hosp Psychiatry 2001 Jul-Aug;23(4):182-92.

5. Speca M; Carlson LE; Goodey E; Angen M. A randomized, wait-list controlled clinical trial: the effect of a mindfulness meditation-based stress reduction program on mood and symptoms of stress in cancer outpatients. Psychosom Med 2000 Sep-Oct;62(5):613-22.

6. Stein, F. Occupation stress, relaxation therapies, exercise and biofeedback. Work 2001; 17(3):235-245.

7. Weil, A. Breathing. (Mark McCoin CD's, 2002)

7

Headache Triggers, Caffeine & Social Support

A Trigger is not the Same Thing as a "Cause" - but it can Certainly Initiate

When a person gets a migraine that is suspected of being brought on by a powerful food or weather trigger, the treating physician accesses what foods they have ingested recently as well as exposure to other triggers, in the hope of identifying a powerful "trigger" that induced the migraine.

Common triggers to "induce" a migraine to a headache sufferer might be red wine, MSG (monosodiumglutamate), aged cheeses, chocolate, and barometric weather conditions, to name a few potential triggers. Getting to know your body and what "sets off" or "triggers" a migraine is very helpful to both the sufferer and the physician.

It is important to mention that if you are a headache sufferer that is prone to bad headaches from time to time - it is wise and economical for you to try and identify the trigger that sets your migraine in motion.

It has often been said that migraine sufferers possess a "faulty nervous system" that is very sensitive to outside triggers. To isolate your trigger and to use trigger-avoidance wherever necessary, will help you cope with your condition.

Sometimes a clear answer to your headache issue, is not immediately possible. The sooner that you accept that you are unfortunately "headache prone" the better off you will be.

Listed below are some usual triggers that you might want to chart – (see Chapter 13, Record Keeping) - but remember that your individual headache pattern may or may not fall under these general guidelines.

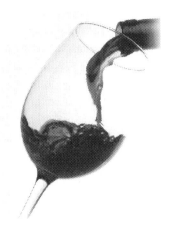

A huge myth that people (either headache sufferers or non-sufferers) make is that caffeine is almost always bad for you. The truth is caffeine could be your trigger and should therefore be avoided at all costs, but very often caffeine can act as a potent vasoconstrictor, thereby helping the sufferer to abort or stop a headache attack. Most over-the-counter headache medicines have caffeine in them for this very reason. See Chapter 7, Caffeine.

Caffeine & Headache
As we Find Out - there is "Good" News & "Bad" News!

Caffeine is a powerful vasoconstrictor that is found in many leaves and plants, and when ingested makes the blood vessels shrink, or constrict - thus aiding to prevent a headache attack. The most common examples of drinks and foods containing caffeine include coffee, tea, cola drinks, some soft drinks, and chocolate.

Many over-the-counter (OTC) medicines contain caffeine as one of their agents. Some examples of OTC's that contain caffeine are: 1) Tylenol #1
   2) 222s
   3) Fiorinal

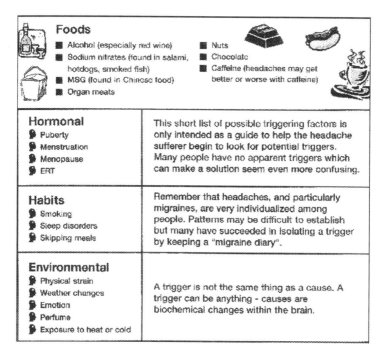

Foods
- Alcohol (especially red wine)
- Sodium nitrates (found in salami, hotdogs, smoked fish)
- MSG (found in Chinese food)
- Organ meats
- Nuts
- Chocolate
- Caffeine (headaches may get better or worse with caffeine)

Hormonal ● Puberty ● Menstruation ● Menopause ● ERT	This short list of possible triggering factors is only intended as a guide to help the headache sufferer begin to look for potential triggers. Many people have no apparent triggers which can make a solution seem even more confusing.
Habits ● Smoking ● Sleep disorders ● Skipping meals	Remember that headaches, and particularly migraines, are very individualized among people. Patterns may be difficult to establish but many have succeeded in isolating a trigger by keeping a "migraine diary".
Environmental ● Physical strain ● Weather changes ● Emotion ● Perfume ● Exposure to heat or cold	A trigger is not the same thing as a cause. A trigger can be anything - causes are biochemical changes within the brain.

So as you can see caffeine can be good but it can also be a "trigger" of migraines, to many sufferers of headache. If ingesting caffeine causes you to have a migraine - then using "trigger-avoidance" would be a wise choice.

CAFFEINE CONTENT OF COMMON FOODS AND DRUGS		
Product	**Example**	**Caffeine** Content (mg)
Tea and Chocolate	Baking Chocolate (1 oz)	35
	Chocolate Candy Bar	25
	Cocoa Beverage (6 oz. mixture)	10
	Milk Chocolate (1 oz.)	6
Coffee	Decaffeinated (5 oz.)	2
	Drip (5 oz.)	146
	Instant, Regular (5 oz.)	53
	Percolated (5 oz.)	110
Over the Counter Drugs	Anacin	32
	Excedrin	65
	No-Doz Tablets	100 200
	Vanquish	33
	Vivarin Tablets	200
Prescription Drugs	Darvon	32.4
	Esgie	40
	Fioiecet	40
	Norgesic	30
	Norgesic Forte	60
	Supac	33
	Synalgos-DC	30
Soft Drinks (12oz)	7-UP/Diet 7-Up	0
	Coca-Cola	34
	Diet Pepsi	34
	Dr. Pepper	38
	Fresca	0
	Ginger Ale	0
	Hires Root Beer	0
	Mountain Dew	52
	Pepsi-Cola	37
	Tab	44
Tea	1-minute brew (5 oz.)	9-33
	3-minute brew (5 oz.)	22-46
	5-minute brew (5 oz.)	20-50
	Canned Ice Tea (12 oz.)	22-36

A Neurologist in Massachusetts writes:

Caffeine & Headache: Good News & Bad News
Reprinted with with permission
by David M. Biondi, D.O. Neurologist
Massachusetts General Hospital
Boston, Massachusetts

Caffeine is a naturally occurring substance found in the leaves, seeds or fruit of more than 60 different plants. Some familiar sources of caffeine include coffee beans, coco beans, kola nuts, and tea leaves. Caffeine is contained in several over-the-counter and prescription pain relievers. The role of caffeine in the cause and treatment of headache is complex and often misunderstood.

The "Good News" is that small amounts of caffeine can help to relieve headaches especially when combined with simple pain relievers. When used in combination with pain relievers, caffeine promotes a more rapid and complete absorption of the pain medicine. Caffeine itself can provide pain relief in some people. Caffeine is a mild brain stimulant and can raise levels of certain brain chemicals which can help relieve the pain and fatigue that is often associated with migraine and other headaches.

The "Bad News" is that caffeine can trigger or worsen headaches when used in excess. Although people can differ greatly in their sensitivity to caffeine, taking more than 300-400 milligrams of caffeine a day (2-3 cups of strong coffee) for several days can worsen headache patterns and cause caffeine toxicity. Excessive caffeine use can cause anxiety, sleeplessness, stomach pain and headache. In addition to the direct triggering of headache after excessive daily caffeine intake, caffeine withdrawal headaches can result whenever the level of caffeine in the blood drops. Headaches which occur mainly on weekends, for example, may be triggered by caffeine withdrawal in a person who drinks a lot of coffee on weekdays while at work.

It is important for people who experience frequent or recurrent headache to remain aware of their daily caffeine intake. If excessive caffeine consumption is present, a gradual reduction of caffeine intake to no more than 200-300 milligrams a day is recommended. Others may attempt a small amount of caffeine when headache occurs as a headache treatment or to enhance the effectiveness of headache medications.

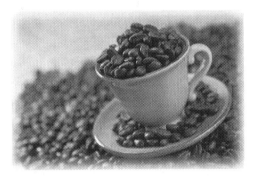

Social Support

Many headache sufferers choose to self-treat themselves by taking large quantities of over-the-counter pain medicines. This notion of "I choose to do it alone", can also be a factor when it comes to avoiding social support.

We all agree in the concept that there is strength in numbers, in any support social situation. Most of us like the fact that we are not alone.
Social support can come in many forms; walking, exercising, support groups and online chat rooms for headache sufferers. Sometimes merely "venting" on the phone - or over a cup of coffee - can really make a difference. The body's pain preventing chemicals are released, which are the endorphins. Endorphins make us "feel good" and often counteract against serotonin, the bodies chemical largely responsible for migraine pain.

Walking is not only good for your circulation, but if you choose to go with a walking partner, you now have added social support for your headaches.

Exercising has long since been an effective way to maintain staying fit, reducing or managing head pain, and it is an effective way to gain better circulation.

Some breathing techniques are helpful too - see Chapter 5 - Alternative Treatments.
Fitness Clubs are great places to foster lasting friendships as well as in consulting with a fitness instructor about how exercise influences your headaches.

Support groups are an effective way to manage any problem, and headache is no exception. The notion is to "draw emotional strength" from others' misfortune. Other members in a support group setting often need an "outlet" for their confusion, frustration, anger, shame, depression, hurt, - the list goes on and on. Many come to realize that they are indirectly a cause of their situation. This, no doubt, adds an element of shame to deal with. But support groups provide that sense of understanding which many situations do not have.

So why all this talk on emotions? Headache pain and emotional pain are highly linked. If the physician advises the patient to try a medicine, but that sufferer refuses to seek help for their emotions, they can be heading for trouble.

The following article is called "What is a Headache Support Group?"

What is a Headache Support Group?
by Brent Lucas
London, Ontario, Canada

People shy away from support groups for a variety of reasons. Actually, they can be a pillar of emotional help and sound knowledge. I will first look at why people stay away, then I will address the reasons why sufferers should attend.

Headache sufferers (or people in general) are very proud creatures. They tend to be private persons and for those reasons alone they can "shy away" from support groups. Another important factor is the "I've tried everything syndrome". Another justification is that they "don't have time...our lives are too busy....we need to work or raise our children."

And let's face it - it does require a monthly, or bimonthly commitment and a few hours is sometimes hard to scrape up. A sufferer would much rather talk to a headache professional on a one-to-one basis, than discuss their feelings and findings within a group format. We have all watched TV shows about stars in rehabilitation, or in a support group, and we can all identify with the "uncomfortableness" that they must feel.

Let's look at the possible reasons to go:

You have to "give it a shot". How can you honestly say that this is not helpful in your situation when you have not gone, nor applied yourself? And go more than once to give yourself a few opportunities to be a part of something worthwhile.

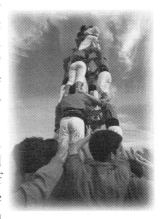

Let's look at the cost factor. Support groups are free and you will usually come home with all kinds of handouts. Your facilitators will line up professional speakers who often bring handouts for reading at a later time.

Caution: As strong as the urge is, a support group facilitator should discourage "cross-talk". As sufferers share in your group you will have a "popcorn of thoughts" going off in your head, as you identify with a person's story. Their story mirrors your own story and you begin to have feelings of empathy for them. Often you begin to feel better and can get lost in a sea of feelings for the other person.

8

Tests, Headache in the Emergency Room, Headaches after Head Injuries and Neck Problems & Headache

online testing helps both sufferers and physicians

Tests

Diagnostic Tests

There is no laboratory or x-ray test that will diagnose the most common causes of headache – tension-type, migraine and cluster headache. The diagnosis is based on clinical grounds, that is, your symptoms and neurologic examination. This is why your doctor asks you many different questions about the location, duration and frequency of your headaches as well as what tends to trigger them (hormonal and weather changes are common examples).

If features in the clinical history or physical examination suggest the possibility that something more ominous is causing the headache, then further investigation is indicated. Imaging can help identify a headache that is caused by something secondary, such as another disease process (see Chapter 3 - Headaches Due to Disease). There are some patients that, despite their physician's reassurance, will not feel reassured about a diagnosis without further testing. The decision to organize testing for patients is up to the discretion of the physician after thorough consultation with the patient; and, so long as there is no added risk to the patient in undergoing that test.

For nearly 30 years, physicians have watched the advances

that have been made in imaging of neural tissues like the brain. Early radiographic techniques to image the human brain were not terribly beneficial since the brain is almost entirely composed of soft tissue that is not radio-opaque. Therefore, it remains essentially invisible to ordinary or plain x-ray examination. The advent of more sophisticated testing such as the CAT scan and MRI have helped physicians obtain more detailed anatomic images of the brain which can be used for diagnostic and research purposes.

Several routine diagnostic tests that are available in most centres are outlined below.

Computerized Tomography (CT) Scan. This imaging test allows your doctor to visualize your brain, in two-dimensional slices. Split-second computer processing creates these images as a series of very thin X-ray beams pass through your body. Sometimes you may have a dye (contrast medium) injected into a vein before the test. The clearer images produced with the dye make it easier to distinguish a tumor or other pathology from normal tissue. A CT scan exposes you to more radiation than do conventional X-rays, but in most cases, the benefits of the test outweigh the risks. Patients should alert their physician to any allergies; rarely,

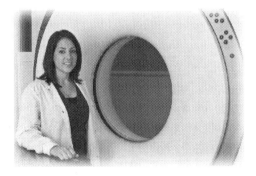

patients can react to the intravenous dye.

Magnetic Resonance Imaging (MRI). With the advancement of MRI imaging, physicians have been able to diagnose many different causes of headache. MRI uses the variation in signals produced by protons in the body when the head is placed in a strong magnetic field. Three-dimensional x-rays of the brain are then produced for assessment by a trained physician. Injection of a dye to enhance the cerebral blood vessels (angiography) may be required to diagnose certain causes of headache (underlying aneurysm).

During the test, you are placed in a small, cylindrical tube that can seem confining to some people. The machine also makes a loud thumping and banging noise. In most cases, you'll be given earplugs to dampen the noise. If you have a history of claustrophobia, your physician can provide you with a mild sedative to allow you to undergo the investigation in a more comfortable manner.

Electroencephalograms (EEG). An EEG is a neurological test that measures the electrical signals within your brain, and records them on a graph. An EEG is used to evaluate the cause of seizures, diagnose comas, and evaluate strokes and sleep disorders. It can also be used to determine the presence and location of brain injuries, abscesses, tumours, bleeding within the brain, and to confirm brain death.

Lumbar Puncture (LP). This procedure (also called a "spinal tap") is used to collect and look at the fluid (cerebrospinal fluid, or CSF) surrounding the brain and spinal cord. During a lumbar puncture, a needle is carefully inserted into the spinal canal low in the back (lumbar area). Samples of CSF are collected. The samples are studied for color, blood cell counts, protein, glucose, and other substances. Some of the sample may be put into a special culture cup to see if any infection grows. The pressure of the CSF also is measured during the procedure. This procedure may be done to a headache patient to diagnose conditions such as meningitis or subarachnoid hemorrhage.

Miscellaneous Tests. Other tests to analyze brain function include PET scanning (Positron Emission Tomography),

SPECT scan (Single Photon Emission Computed Tomography) or FMRI (Functional MRI). None of these tests is used to diagnose primary headache disorders such as migraine.

reviewed by Dr. Ian Finkelstein, M.Sc., M.D., D.A.A.P.M.
Board Certified, American Academy of Pain Management
Director, Toronto Headache & Pain Clinic
Neurologist with interest in headache

Online Tests

There has been a recent interest in doing online tests so that sufferers use these online assessment tools and then follow-up with their physician. The following article describes online assessment testing.

Do you want to learn more about your headaches using online assessment tools?
Reprinted with permission from the World Headache Alliance website - www.w-h-a.org

40 people participated in the poll

> **"Yes!"** was the response of **36** people
> **"No, I'm not interested"** was the response of **1** person
> **"I have already used them"** was the response of **3** people

Everyone who suffers from headaches can benefit from learning more about their headaches so they can seek the appropriate treatment.

There are two excellent headache management tools available to help you understand your headaches and how they are affecting your life: the **Headache Impact Test (HIT)** and the **Migraine Disability Assessment Questionnaire (MIDAS)**.

The **Headache Impact Test**, or HIT, is a tool to measure the impact headaches have on a person's ability to function on the job, at home, at school and in social situations. From your score on a 1 to 2 minute questionnaire, HIT will provide you with an extremely accurate description of the impact headaches are having on your life and your ability to function. You can use these results when discussing your headaches with your doctor, so that he/she can better understand the impact they are having on your life.

The HIT test has been proven to be valid by headache experts and is the most reliable method for evaluating an individual patient's progress over time.

For the Headache Impact Test (HIT) go to www.headachetest.com

The **Migraine Disability Assessment (MIDAS) Questionnaire** was first developed to improve migraine care by helping physicians to identify sufferers most severely affected by their migraine and, therefore, most in need of care. The MIDAS approach increases the likelihood of patients receiving the most effective treatment, the first time they visit their physician about migraine.

MIDAS measures headache-related disability. Five questions count the number of days of lost or limited activity due to migraine. Activities are classed into three domains:

• Paid work and education (school/college)

• Household work (unpaid work such as housework, shopping, and taking care of children and others)

• Non-work activities (family, social and leisure activities)

The overall MIDAS score (expressed as a number of days) is obtained by summing the answers to the questions.

The MIDAS questionnaire provides a basis for patients to discuss their illness with their physician and how their headaches are really affecting their lives.

Using the MIDAS grading system, physicians can quickly assess the medical needs of their patients, and prescribe appropriate treatment at the first consultation. MIDAS, can also help physicians gauge whether referral to a specialist is needed. Similarly, it can help medical professionals decide whether patients should consult their physician.

MIDAS can be used by anyone suffering from headaches. It can be completed alone, or in the company of a healthcare professional such as a pharmacist, nurse practitioner, family practitioner or specialist. It can be used at the initial consultation, and then throughout the treatment period to monitor progress.

MIDAS has been rigorously tested for reliability and validity in clinical and research settings.

Take a few minutes and see how your headaches rate on the HIT and MIDAS scores. And then discuss your results at your next doctor appointment so that you can get the treatment that is best for you.

> *For the Migraine Disability Assessment (MIDAS)*
> *Questionnaire go to:*
> *www.midas-migraine.net*

Editor's note: Both of these online headache tests are in alternate languages.

Emergency Room

Treatment of Acute Head Pain in the Emergency Room
by Robert L. Hamel, Pa-C
Michigan Headache & Neurological Institute,
Ann Arbor, Michigan

The assessment and treatment of head pain in an emergency department or other urgent care setting is common but can become complicated in some situations:

1) This is the first or worst headache of a person's life.

2) The person's visit to the emergency department is part of a pattern of regular use of emergency service department services for the treatment of head pain.

3) The person is in a toxic or otherwise drug dependent state.

4) The person is suffering from dehydration or other metabolic condition which if left untreated would compromise the person's health.

5) There is a concurrent medical illness which could be causing head pain or limiting the effectiveness of headache treatment.

The usual reason a person seeks treatment in an emergency department for pain is the occasional acute, severe attack of migraine that has been ineffectively treated at home. In this situation, allowing for the person's sensitivities and allergies to medication, there are many treatment options.

Before looking at treatment options certain other conditions need to be considered. The first and/or worst headache must always be assumed to be something other than migraine or other benign headache until proven otherwise. The first or worst headache requires that the emergency department physician rule out the possibility of an intra-cranial hemorrhage or other significant medical/neurological cause of headache such as meningitis.

The emergency department physician is also wary of a person who uses the emergency department regularly for treatment of headache. This could indicate a dependence on regular injections of narcotic medication, which could be part of a pattern of medication overuse headache. Patients presenting with this type of problem should be referred to a primary care physician after acute treatment. Establishing a plan of care that will significantly limit the need for emergency department treatment of head pain is the goal.

Treatment of a medical illness such as sinusitis may result in complete resolution of headache. Other illnesses may be more difficult to uncover, but eventually lead to proper treatment and pain relief.

If a person is dehydrated due to nausea and vomiting and/or diarrhea associated with migraine headache, overnight hospitalization may be required. There are many treatment options available. The following medications are listed with examples of each.

1) **Dihydroergotamine-45** (DHE-45) is the injectable form of ergot medication that is often used in the emergency department. This medication is generally safe, though it should be avoided in people with significant cardiac and vascular risk factors.

2) **Triptans:** Sumatriptan (Imitrex) is readily available to many outpatients. For some people who had not had this medication, the emergency department setting may be a good opportunity to use this medication for the first time. Other forms and types of this medication come in an oral form and nasal spray. (Warning - significant cardiac adverse effects can occur when using this type of medication. Persons receiving this type of medication should be screened for cardiovascular risk factors).

3) **Opioid** (narcotic) medication: This group of medications can be effective and relatively free of adverse effects in the appropriate person when not used too regularly. Such medications as meperidine (Demerol), morphine and nalbuphine (Nubain) can all be very effective. Cautions include the avoidance of Demerol in people with a history of seizure disorder.

4) **Nonsteroidal anti-inflammatory drugs:** An injectable medication useful in an emergency department setting is ketorolac, taken intramuscularly. People should avoid this medication if there is a history of peptic ulcer disease, kidney disease, or colitis.

5) **Another category of medication is the neuroleptic.** These medications are also very effective anti-nauseants and include chlorpromazine and promethazine.

6) **Antihistamines:** Of the category hydroxyzine, taken intramuscularly, can provide both some pain relief as well as reduction in nausea. Diphenhydramine can be used intravenously or intramuscularly at doses ranging from 25-75 mg.

It is important to note that this is an American article and medications may not be available - or go under a different name.

Please consult your physician or neurologist.

In summary, the treatment of head pain in the emergency department is common and usually uncomplicated. When there is medical complication, treatment of pain must sometimes be delayed until diagnostic tests are done. Treatment of acute severe headache, most often migrainous, is carried out by using a variety of different medications. An accurate and detailed history is necessary to be sure that the safest and most effective treatment is provided.

Headaches after Head Injuries (or Post-Traumatic Headaches)

Headaches After Head Injuries - Post-Traumatic Headaches
reprinted with permission
by Seymour Solomon, MD. - Headache Unit
Montefiore Medical Center
Albert Einstein College of Medicine
New York, NY

Headache immediately following a head injury usually clears after minutes or days but sometimes headaches may persist for months or rarely for years. The long term headaches are called post-traumatic or post concussion headaches.

One can understand why headaches may follow a moderate or severe injury to the brain such as a concussion (bruise) or laceration (tear). What has been more difficult to understand and has presented an ongoing controversy are chronic headaches following mild head injuries.

Mild injuries to the brain are characterized as a concussion (a brief disturbance of brain functioning causing loss of consciousness or transient difficulty in thought processes). Because the neurological examination after mild head injury is normal and standard tests as well as imaging studies (such as MRI or CT of the head) similarly fail to reveal abnormalities, many thought that the symptoms following mild head injury were psychological.

But microscopic studies have shown disruption of the nerve fibers in the brain due to the stretching or shearing forces of the trauma. Other subtle changes have been noted in brain functioning.

The clinical features of post-traumatic headache may vary from one individual to another. Most headaches would be now classified as chronic tension-type headache. These headaches are typically a steady ache affecting both sides of the head and occurring daily or almost everyday. They are of slight to moderate intensity but intermittently, upon this base of low grade headache, bouts of severe or moderately severe headache may occur and these often are similar to, if not identical with migraine (one-sided throbbing pain associated with nausea and sensitivity to light and noise).

Unfortunately, people who experience post-traumatic headaches also experience other symptoms of the post-traumatic or post-concussion syndrome. There may be other neurological symptoms such as dizziness, ringing-of-the-ears, vague blurring of vision; psychological symptoms occur such as depression, anxiety, personality change, disturbances in sleep - (see www.headache-help.org - free articles - Sleep Disorders & Headache) - and impairment libido.

Finally, people with the post-concussion syndrome have changes in their mental functioning, primarily difficulty in concentration, inability to work effectively and associated difficulty maintaining attention and retaining memory.

The treatment of post-traumatic headache, as well as other features of the post-traumatic syndrome is symptomatic. That is each symptom is treated individually because, unfortunately, there is no medication that will alter the underlying disturbance in the brain.

Most often treatment of the chronic tension-type headache consists of such medications as the tricyclic antidepressants (for example amitriptyline). These agents not only diminish depression but also decrease pain.

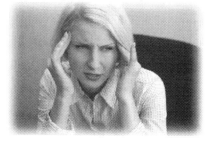

The periodic worsening of headaches, if they have characteristics of migraine, are treated with typical migraine medications (for example sumatriptan for an acute attack).

Non-drug methods of therapy are also advisable. Healthy habits should be encouraged by elimination of nicotine and alcohol, by recommendations for regularity with regard to sleep and meal time and by exercise at least every other day. Relaxation techniques may be helpful. These can be learned by techniques as well as by such methods as biofeedback.

Last but not least is attention to psychological factors. The family, friends and employer or teacher should be educated to the fact that headaches are not purely psychological but have a basis related to the disturbed structure and chemical functions of the brain. A psychologist may be helpful in teaching pain coping techniques and in treating the psychological symptoms that are part of the post-traumatic syndrome.

Fortunately, most headaches following head injury gradually taper off within the first 3 to 6 months. Even those unfortunate individuals who experience symptoms much longer can be helped.

Neck Problems & Headache
reprinted with permission
by Seymour Solomon, MD. -
Headache Unit
Montefiore Medical Center
Albert Einstein College of
Medicine
New York, NY

There is no doubt that serious disease of the neck (cervical spine) may cause pain not only in the neck but extending to all parts of the head. Such conditions as a fractured vertebrae or a large herniated disk are common examples of serious problems. More often pain in the neck and the head is not associated with obvious disease that can be seen on examination or in imaging studies of the neck. The most common examples are whiplash injuries associated with rear-end motor vehicle accident. The whiplashing effect of the neck may cause injury to the muscle and ligaments of the neck, but there are no standard tests to evaluate these so-called soft tissue injuries.

The mechanism of pain is very complex. There are a number of things that can modify pain. The brain may produce certain pain-suppressing chemicals, called endorphins, that dampen the experience of pain and the brain may send signals down the nervous system to suppress the impulses of pain that are coming up to the brain. Some people appear to have severe and prolonged pain after a relatively minor injury and others may have slight and only brief pain after severe injury. For example, a soldier wounded in battle may not experience pain until the battle is over.

In the United States, Canada and England, pain following whiplash injuries often persists for months or years. In Lithuania, Greece and Germany, however, chronic pain following whiplash injury is very rare. How can there be such a wide discrepancy in the occurrence of chronic whiplash neck and head pain?

Cultural and social factors play an important role in the experience of pain. Just the expectation of pain may heighten its intensity and duration. On the other hand, if there is no expectation of pain and the injury is limited to soft tissues, there is a very strong chance that prolonged chronic pain will not occur. Chronic whiplash symptoms are rare in children, athletes and demolition car drivers because they have no expectation of long lasting pain. People in Lithuania and Greece do not expect to have prolonged pain after a whiplash injury. They are encouraged to return to work and resume normal activities as soon as possible. In the United States, Canada and England, on the other hand, just the opposite is often recommended. People know about chronic whiplash pain; their physicians, chiropractors, physical therapists and lawyers anticipate a chronic problem. And this expectation is in fact realized in a high percentage of people involved in motor vehicle accidents in

North America and England.

In summary, the best way to avoid chronic pain after you have been rear-ended (and have been assured that there is no fracture or herniation) is to return to work and normal activities as soon as possible.

9

Chronic Daily Headache, (includes Medication Overuse), Fibromyalgia & Chronic Fatigue Syndrome

Is my headache a Chronic Daily Headache?

Often, sufferers say that they are not absolutely sure if they have a headache or a migraine. This can be a very frustrating area for both the sufferer who is looking for answers and also for the treating physician.

Many times, a sufferer will begin with what sounds like a tension-type headache; then eventually will complain of bouts of migrainous headaches with nausea.

You should also be aware of the fact that medicines used to treat tension headaches also treat some migraine headaches.

If you are confused if you have either tension-type or migraine, ask yourself:

- Do I have symptoms of tension headaches that include spikes of migraine in them?

- Have I looked into the symptoms of a Chronic Daily Headache? See below on Chronic Daily Headache article.

- Did my migraines evolve from tension headaches?

- Do I take lots of over-the-counter pain medicine?

- Does my migraine medication reduce my tension headaches?

Chronic Daily Headache
By Christine Lay, MD, FRCP
Director, Women's College Hospital Centre For Headache
Women's College Hospital
Toronto, Canada

Headache is a problem of enormous scope, affecting individuals across all socioeconomic backgrounds, with a lifetime prevalence of 93-99%. It is one of the most common ailments in the primary care physician's office and is a costly, disabling public health problem, both for the individual and for society.

Despite headache being such a widespread problem, patients are often misdiagnosed, mismanaged or are attempting to manage their headaches with over-the-counter medications. Patients with chronic daily headache (CDH) are especially difficult to diagnose and manage, as these are often difficult to classify. The International Headache Society (IHS) has developed explicit criteria for many headache disorders; however CDH remains incompletely defined. Classification is further complicated by the fact that CDH is often associated with overuse of pain relievers (analgesics) or often coexists with other disorders such as depression or anxiety. For the purpose of this article, CDH will refer to primary headaches (not secondary to another cause such as a brain tumour or medical illness), lasting four or more hours, occurring more than 15 days per month.

Diagnosis

Proper diagnoses is essential to ensure appropriate treatment. The term CDH can be divided into four types: chronic/transformed migraine, chronic tension-type headache, new daily persistent headache and hemicrania continua. All of these headache types may or may not be associated with medication overuse. The majority of patients falls into the chronic migraine category. The exact cause of CDH remains unknown. Excessive use of pain medications (analgesics) may promote chronicity of headache and external factors related to physical, psychological stress, trauma, or illness and may affect the nervous system, perhaps reducing the brain's natural pain controlling mechanisms. Up to 20% of CDH's are daily from the onset and the remaining 80% appear to evolve from episodic headaches.

Chronic Migraine/Transformed Migraine

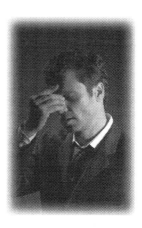

Episodic migraine may evolve or transform to a more chronic or daily pattern; however, it may be difficult or impossible to pinpoint exactly when this transformation took place. In addition to the daily mild to moderate head or face pain, patients usually continue to experience superimposed attacks of episodic migraine. Overuse of medication may or may not play a role in the perpetuation of this headache; however, nearly 80% of cases are associated with excessive use of analgesics.

Chronic Tension-Type Headache

Chronic tension-type headache (CTTH) is similar to episodic tension-type headache except for frequency. Nausea as well as light and sound intolerance may be associated with CTTH. The headache is generally described as a bilateral pressure or tight feeling "headache" that is of mild or moderate severity.

New Daily Persistent Headache

Patients suffering with new daily persistent headache (NDPH) often recall the exact time and date of onset of the headache. It often develops over three days and occasionally follows a viral illness. There is no prior history of migraine or tension-type headache in these patients. The headache is described as an unremitting head pain, localized to one specific region of the head. On average, the headache occurs more than 15 days per month and lasts more than 4 hours per day.

Hemicrania Continua

Hemicrania continua (HC), while a rare headache disorder, is an important headache of which to be aware, due to its unique and impressive response to a drug called **Indomethacin.** HC is described as a continuous, baseline, mild to moderate pain, localized to one side of the head, with superimposed attacks of more severe stabbing-like pain. These attacks may last minutes to days and are occasionally associated with same-side "automatic" features such as tearing and redness of the eye, droopy eyelid, running nose and nasal congestion. HC may occasionally follow head trauma.

Treatment

Keeping a diary of headaches, noting time of day, potential aggravating/alleviating factors and analgesic use is often helpful. A review of this diary will help identify provoking factors that can be eliminated and, more importantly, it will determine if medication overuse is a contributing factor (see Diary - Chapter 13 - How to Prepare for Your Physician's Appointment). Non-pharmacologic treatments such as biofeedback, acupuncture and relaxation therapy play an important role in addition to acute and preventative therapies. Maintaining regular eating and sleeping patterns as well as regular exercise is critical.

If your diary reveals use of over-the-counter or prescription medication use more than two days per week, you are at risk of developing rebound headache. Medication Overuse Headache (formerly rebound headache) is characterized by a predictable pattern of escalating use of headache medication associated with an increasing frequency of headache and decreasing effectiveness of medication. Commonly overused pain medications include acetaminophen, ibuprofen, aspirin-caffeine-acetaminophen combinations, butalbital-containing drugs and even triptans. The most important aspect of treatment in this case is discontinuation of the medication; without this step, you are unlikely to improve. While tapering off the medication, you may experience a worsening of headaches; however, improvement is usually noted within four to six weeks but may take several months. During this "withdrawal" period, a short course of a preventative agent (a tricyclic antidepressant, a beta-blocker or an anticonvulsant) and headache medications are usually helpful.

Preventative Therapy

A number of medications are helpful in the treatment of CDH with the choice often depending on the presence or absence of other medical conditions. It is important to note that preventative therapy may take weeks to months to become fully effective, during which time adjustments of doses and/or changes in medications may be required. A realistic goal of therapy is to reduce headache frequency and severity, rather than to eliminate all headaches. In general, medications should be started at low doses and slowly titrated upward to minimize side-effects and to avoid excess dosing. As patients are highly variable in their responses to medications, it is worthwhile trying more than one drug in any particular class. Most of these medications are not specifically approved for headache prevention.

When single agent therapy fails, combination therapy is often effective. If you feel you are unable or unwilling to discontinue analgesics in the outpatient setting, a short course of hospitalization, perhaps for intravenous DHE 45 (dihydroergotamine) may be required to "break the cycle". Then you are referred to a specialty center.

Botulinum toxin is a new agent in the headache armamentarium and is beginning to show promise as an effective agent in the prevention of some chronic or frequent headaches. It requires injections every three months but overall has quite a good response rate.

115

If you are experiencing headaches more than 15 days per months, you may have chronic daily headaches and should seek the guidance and help of your physician. Without careful supervision or assistance from medications one-third of patients may relapse and begin analgesic use. However, with perseverance on the part of both yourself and your physician, effective treatment of CDH can be achieved.

Medication Overuse Headaches
Previously called Medication-Induced Headaches or Rebound Headaches.

Medication Overuse Headaches are often caused by a condition where, over time, pain relievers which used to stop headaches - now cause more frequent and/or severe headaches. It is the concept of ""too much of a good thing"". Overuse of medication such as narcotics (Percocets, Vicodan), barbiturate combination drugs (Fioricet, Esgic), caffeine-containing drugs (Excedrin, Tylenol 1, 2 & 3, Anacin), vasoconstricting medications (Ergotamine, Cafergot) or even decongestants (Sudafed), may escalate headache frequency in certain individuals. Medication overuse headaches have been termed the "silent epidemic" because it is often under-recognized and under-diagnosed. Patients, as well as health care professionals, may overlook this condition as a cause for headaches, and this can lead to ineffective and frustrating courses of treatment.

"Overuse" should not be confused with "Headache Recurrence". If a pain-relieving medication is cleared out of the body quickly, and the headache mechanism is still present, the headache may recur. Even newer effective medications, such as Imitrex, have a recurrence rate of 40% within 24 hours of the initial dose.

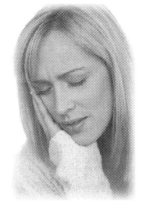

Self-treatment of headaches with over-the-counter medications is the norm for most headache sufferers. Most migraine or tension-type headache sufferers do not consult a health care professional for diagnosis or treatment. Over-the-counter medication may "get them by" and allow functioning with headaches but usually it is not the most effective treatment regimen available. Development of medication overuse headaches with the overuse of these medications, as well as loss of effectiveness over time may prompt the sufferer to use higher than recommended doses which may affect the stomach, liver or kidneys.

Caffeine is a common offender in medication overuse headaches. Coffee, tea, cola and beverages such as Mountain Dew and orange soda may contain caffeine. Caffeine is an ingredient on some over-the-counter and prescription medications. Caffeine speeds absorption of medication in the stomach and gives a pain-relieving "boost" to many drugs. Taken in limited quantities, caffeine can be an effective "drug". See Chapter 7 - Caffeine.

However, using caffeinated beverages or medications more frequently than two days in a week may be a set-up for more headaches. It is the frequency of medication use (number of days per week) rather than the amount of pills used that is the important factor. For example, you are less likely to get medication overuse headaches if you use 6 Fioricet only two days per week rather than using 1 Fioricet everyday of the week. Near-daily use of pain relievers may change levels of brain chemicals over time, making you more prone to "setting off" headaches.

Patients most likely to get medication overuse headaches are those who get more than one type of headache. Some headache sufferers start with infrequent migraine headaches, and then develop milder tension-type headaches that gradually become more frequent and lead to more frequent medication use. This may lead to what is termed "transformed migraine" or "chronic daily headache" where patients get near-daily headaches with a mixture of both migraine and tension-type headache symptoms.

These patients often lose the ability to distinguish between the different types of headaches and frequently use rebound-causing medications at the first onset of a headache, fearing escalation of pain to a disabling migraine. Medications may eventually lose effectiveness despite higher doses, but patients will still use it because they "need to try something". **The thought of discontinuing these pain killers and worsening headaches can cause much anxiety.**

Treatment involves discontinuing the rebound causing medication. Sixty percent of individuals improve with this measure alone. In most cases, a daily preventative medication would be prescribed to reduce the frequency and severity of headaches. It is important to understand that unless the daily caffeine and pain killers are stopped, the preventative medications will not be effective. The first two weeks of this transition are a trying time, and patients should be prepared for increased headaches. Certainly, some other pain medication would be prescribed during this time, but it may just "take the edge off" and not work as well as the medication overuse-causing medicine. It is tempting to go back to the rebounding medication because it seems the "only thing that works" during this period and daily preventive medication may take several weeks to become fully effective. While most patients are able to "stick it out" and note improvement with out-patient therapy as early as two weeks, some patients may require hospitalization to discontinue these medications. In-patient treatment should take place in a headache treatment unit, not a detox program for addicts. Most medication overuse headache sufferers are not drug addicts. They use medication for pain control and to maintain function in their lives. It is often the absence of appropriate effective treatment that causes patients to resort to overuse of medications.

If you believe you may have medication overuse headaches, it is important to consult a health care provider. A proper diagnosis should be made, and more serious causes of headaches ruled out. You should also be counseled on how to discontinue the rebound-causing medication. In some cases, it may be dangerous to stop the medication abruptly because of the possibility of withdrawal symptoms, including seizures. There is some variation in treatment recommendations, with some headache experts "weaning" medication and others stopping them "cold turkey", believing that the agony of increased headaches is prolonged with weaning a drug. Allow your health care provider to discuss the best individualized treatment regimen for you.

Editors Note: Often, Medication Overuse Headache pain can be felt on the top of the head and can be present upon waking, but this is not always the case.

Please, also remember that this is an American article and medicines might be different…consult a physician, hopefully that specializes in Headaches.

Chronic Daily Headache and Migraine May Result from Sleep Apnea.
Reprinted with permission from the World Headache Alliance website – www.w-h-a.org

The Dartmouth Medical School in New Hampshire and the Johns Hopkins School of Public Health in Baltimore conducted two independent studies to investigate the association between frequent headache and sleep apnea. The Dartmouth study (826 patients) showed that 67% of patients tested who complained of frequent morning headache were found to have sleep apnea, a disorder which causes the person to stop breathing while sleeping, for periods of ten seconds or longer. Eighty-one percent of the total number of patients tested had sleep apnea, which can cause sleep deprivation, possibly exacerbating migraine or chronic headache.

In the Johns Hopkins study, 206 people with chronic daily headache (headache on at least 180 days/year) and 507 people suffering from the average number of headaches (2/month) were then asked how often they snored. Twenty-four percent of those patients with chronic daily headache, who knew they snored were habitual snorers, compared to 14% of those without chronic daily headache who knew if they snored.

The researchers concluded that people with chronic daily headache were about 2.5 times more likely to snore regularly than were people without chronic daily headache. "Yet, when assessing patients with chronic headache, doctors may not routinely ask about snoring or sleep problems", says Ann Scher, PHd, head of the Johns Hopkins study. From: Clinician Reviews 11(11):85-90, 2001.

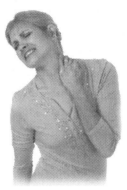

Fibromyalgia & Headache and Chronic Fatigue Syndrome
Reprinted with permission from the Michigan Headache & Neurological Institute website, Ann Arbor, Michigan.

What is fibromyalgia?

Fibromyalgia is a condition involving painful muscles, ligaments, and tendons. It is not disfiguring or life threatening or progressive (i.e., does not necessarily worsen over time). It is not related to tissue inflammation like arthritis. Similar to migraine headache, fibromyalgia affects mostly women in middle age, and less often affects children and the elderly.

The pain from fibromyalgia may occur in four or more distinct areas of the body, and may be related to distinct "trigger points". "Trigger points" or "tender points" in the body can affect pain and muscle spasm when pressure is applied. Trigger points are often found in the elbows, shoulders, back of the head, knees, and the sides of the breast bone. The presence of widespread pain and trigger points, occurring for three or more months, is necessary for the diagnosis of fibromyalgia. Migraine headache is a common associated problem. Other associated symptoms include fatigue, sleep disturbance (especially feeling tired in the morning after a night's sleep), depressed and anxious mood, poor concentration and memory, and gastrointestinal symptoms such as spastic colon.

In July 1996 the National Institute of Health sponsored a scientific workshop entitled "The Neuroscience and Endocrinology of Fibromyalgia". The latest scientific findings on fibromyalgia were presented by prominent medical researchers. One goal of the workshop was to inform the public of sophisticated research which is identifying the causes of fibromyalgia and to stimulate other scientists to do this research. Fibromyalgia may be related to brain chemical changes resulting in abnormalities in the central pain process and disturbances in biological rhythms such as sleep cycles.

Recently, at MHNI's monthly Multidisciplinary Meeting, Drs. Biondi and Silverman updated clinical staff on the current methods of diagnosis and treatment of fibromyalgia. Because the causes of fibromyalgia are not known, there is no cure, but effective treatments have been identified. Dr. Biondi stated that "a graduated stretching, exercise and fitness program may be a critical treatment intervention. A variety of medications have been shown to be effective in controlling the symptoms and can be prescribed. I also instruct patients to improve dietary and sleep habits and consider learning biofeedback skills. With a positive attitude and proper therapy most people suffering from fibromyalgia can improve and lead a productive, active life."

Is there a relationship between chronic fatigue syndrome, fibromyalgia, and migraine headaches?

Many patients with fibromyalgia suffer from migraine-like headaches. It is currently believed that fibromyalgia may be the result of disturbances in the brain's "pain center," a theory very similar to that which explains migraine. In fact, there are many who believe that chronic pain disorders, including migraine and fibromyalgia, may arise from the same type of disturbance. Though the pain of fibromyalgia is frequently found throughout the body, it is associated with a variety of other symptoms, including sleep disturbance, depression, anxiety, and headaches. Migraine is associated with many of these symptoms as well. Many patients who are successfully treated for migraine find that their fibromyalgia is improved.

Chronic fatigue syndrome remains an uncertain clinical entity. Many believe that it is due to a virus that affects the central nervous system which can produce a variety of symptoms which overlap migraine and fibromyalgia. This includes pain, depression, sleep disturbance, and of course recurrent and persistent fatigue. If it is a virus, then it is likely that the virus affects the production of neurotransmitters or their connecting sites (the receptors) on brain cells. Thus, the brain malfunctions, and the symptoms of fatigue, pain, depression, and sleep disturbance develop. Some authorities believe that low blood pressure accounts for its symptoms. Because depression, headaches, and sleep disturbance are common to chronic fatigue, fibromyalgia, and migraine, there may well be overlap in the origin of these. Much more must be known, however, before a definitive solution is available.

10

Hormones & Women with Headache

Why Are Women in their Child-Bearing Years more Prone to Headaches?

It is no secret that the majority of sufferers are female. Why? The powerful female hormone "estrogen" is to blame as it aligns itself with serotonin, the brain chemical largely responsible for migraine. We know that serotonin causes blood vessels to dilate, eventually, sometimes leading to a migraine.

It is of no surprise that migraine tends to peak in females in their child-bearing years, when estrogen is also high.

Below are sections listed on: menstrual migraine, acute therapy, preventative therapy, hormone prophylaxis, headache in pregnancy, oral contraceptive use, menopause and estrogen replacement therapy in menopause.

A Headache Neurologist writes:

Women's Issues in Headache
By Christine Lay, MD, FRCP
Director, Women's College Hospital Centre for Headache
Toronto, Ontario, Canada

Prior to puberty, migraine occurs with a slightly higher frequency in boys than girls, but by age eleven, a female predominance emerges and is quite evident by age 13-15. This female predominance to migraine is directly caused by menarche during puberty and which exists all throughout the female child-bearing years. At menarche the female to male ratio is 3:1 with millions of women affected. Some women will experience a discontinuation of their headaches at menopause and the prevalence again becomes equal in both sexes, falling again in women. The stale old joke of "I can't wait until I pass through menopause - sometimes is applied here".

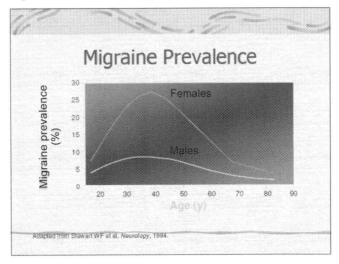

Migraine prevalence is increased in the child-bearing years due to influences of hormonal changes associated with the menstrual cycle, pregnancy, and the birth control pill.

There are many times in a woman's life when hormonal fluctuations may trigger, worsen or bring relief from migraine headache. These include puberty, menstruation, pregnancy, menopause and during oral contraceptive use or hormone replacement therapy. It is unlikely that hormones explain the entire variability of migraine in women, but considerable evidence does exist to suggest that there is a link between migraine and the female estrogenic hormones. The biological basis, however, is not completely understood.

Menstrual Migraine

In women, migraine onset is most frequently in the second decade of life, around puberty, peaking around age forty and thereafter declining, corresponding with menopause.

Unfortunately, menstrual migraine has not been clearly defined nor has the term been used consistently. Menstrual Migraine is referred to as MM and the term menstrually associated migraine (MAM) has been chosen to describe migraine that is exacerbated around the time of menses, but also occurs at other times. Perhaps up to 60% of women migraineurs experience MM.

A smaller number of women, 14%, experience migraine exclusively in the perimenstrual period. This group is said to have true menstrual migraine (TMM). Generally, MM is defined as migraine occurring from two days prior to menses, to 3 days after the onset of menses; the most common day of attack being the first day of menses.

The biochemical mechanism underlying MM has been studied previously, evaluating both estrogens and progesterone as potential targets for triggers. Previous research has shown that there appears to be no difference or abnormalities in hormone levels in migraineurs. It is the fall in estrogen just prior to a woman's period that is believed to be the primary trigger for migraine.

The therapeutic approach to MM is the same as the approach to other migraine attacks. The first step in management is keeping a headache diary, for 3 months (See - How to Prepare for Your Physician's Appointment? - chapter 13.) in which one notes the days on which headache is experienced, timing of menstrual flow and any identifiable triggers. This helps to determine the association, if any, between the migraine attacks and the timing of the menstrual cycle. Non-pharmacological treatments should also be stressed, including avoidance of known triggers, sleep hygiene (keeping "wake up" and "to bed" times consistent weekdays and weekends), good hydration, regular meals and non-medical therapies like biofeedback, relaxation therapy, and acupuncture. In the majority of cases, however, pharmacological intervention is necessary.

Acute Therapy

Anti-nausea drugs are often helpful as these medications often relieve not only the nausea and vomiting associated with migraine, but the headache pain as well. Women with MM need to carefully avoid overuse of analgesic medications - like simple over-the-counter pain medications or prescription drugs like "triptans". Prescription anti-inflammatory medications are often effective in the acute treatment of MM because of their effects on prostaglandins.

Prostaglandins comprise hormone-like substances that participate in a wide range of body functions such as the contraction and relaxation of smooth muscle, the dilation and constriction of blood vessels, control of blood pressure. They are partially responsible for blood vessel dilation, which causes pain and so they deserve being mentioned here.

Narcotic drugs should be tried as a last resort, due to their addictive potential. All of the migraine specific drugs, the "triptans", are efficacious in treating MM. Early intervention is key as is appropriate dosing. As they are available in oral tablet, oral dissolving, nasal spray, and injectable, numerous options are available to women with MM. Once a woman approaches menopausal age (see Online Interview at www.headache-help. org - Q# 7- click on the interview picture in the middle of our homepage), it is critical to review potential cardiovascular risk factors.

Ergotamine drugs are most effective when used early in the course of the migraine attack. Ergotamine preparations are available in oral, sublingual and rectal suppository formulations. Nausea is a common side-effect of ergotamine, which may require pre-dosing with an anti-nausea drug. Caffeine has been combined with ergotamine in some preparations to enhance absorption and may act synergistically with the ergotamine. Dihydroergotamine, available intravenously and in a nasal spray, has been proven effective.

Preventative Therapy

For women experiencing 3-4 or more debilitating headaches per month, preventative therapy may also be required. The goals of preventative therapy are to reduce the frequency, duration and intensity of the migraine headaches. Standard migraine prophylactic medications, such as B-blockers, calcium channel blockers, antidepressants or anticonvulsants, may be used for 3-5 days prior to the onset of menses and continued through to the end of menses. For women who also suffer with migraine at other times of the month and are already taking preventative agents, transiently increasing the dose of their daily medications during the perimenstrual period, often eliminates the menstrual migraine.

Short-term prophylaxis with non-steroidal anti-inflammatories, sumatriptan (Imitrex) and naratriptan (Amerge) - please see Q# 8 - online interview at www.headache-help.org (click on picture) - just before and during a woman's period can be effective options. The exact mechanism of effectiveness is unknown, but theoretically could relate to the prevention of neurogenic inflammation.

Both riboflavin (400mg/day) and magnesium (360mg/day) have been used with some success and may be worth trying in women who prefer "non-drug" therapy. While their efficacy has been demonstrated in recent studies, the benefit is likely small. Side-effects may include diarrhea.

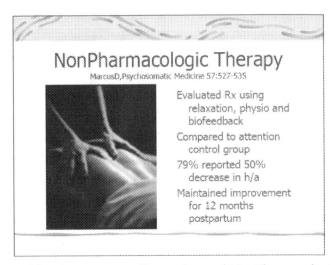

NonPharmacologic Therapy
MarcusD,Psychosomatic Medicine 57:527-535

Evaluated Rx using relaxation, physio and biofeedback

Compared to attention control group

79% reported 50% decrease in h/a

Maintained improvement for 12 months postpartum

79% of female migraine sufferers who used NonPharmacological Therapy - reported a 50% decrease in their headaches.

For those patients with chronic or frequent migraine, botulinum toxin A (Botox A) has been shown to be an effective, safe prophylactic agent. It may reduce frequency, severity and or duration of headaches. Injections are given every three months and effects may be cumulative with repeated treatments.

Hormonal Prophylaxis

Hormonal therapy may be tried for MM resistant to the methods described above, provided there are no contraindications to estrogen therapy. Estrogen use in migraineurs (particularly those who experience migraine with aura) is controversial due to a small but significant increased risk for stroke. Recently, The International Headache Society Task Force on Combined Oral Contraceptives and Hormone Replacement Therapy, concluded that there is no contradiction to the use of OCP's in women with migraine in the absence of migraine aura or other risk factors. Caution should be used in prescribing estrogens to migraineurs with other risk factors for arterial disease, such as smoking, hypertension or diabetes. When prescribing estrogens, choose the lowest possible estrogen dose that is effective. If possible, consultation with the patient's gynecologist or primary care physician is recommended. Additionally, the possibility that the migraines may be worsened, rather than helped by the estrogens, should be known to the patient.

The patient should have menstrual cycles at regular intervals since therapy begins several days prior to menses. The goal of therapy is to stabilize estrogen levels, through hormonal manipulation. Due to variable absorption, oral estrogens typically provide unstable plasma levels and are therefore not generally effective. However, some women have benefited from oral contraception used for three continuous cycles. Transdermal therapy is usually most effective. These methods help to prevent the decline in the level of estrogen.

No long term or controlled studies have been undertaken evaluating hysterectomy in the treatment of MM. Anecdotal reports of success are complicated by the post-operative use of daily estrogen replacement, which may account for the positive results. At present, there is no role for hysterectomy in the management of MM.

Oral Contraceptive Use

Oral contraceptive (OC) use may be associated with worsening of migraine, alleviation of migraine or a triggering of the first attack. In most women, the headache pattern does not change significantly. Pre-existing migraine is frequently exacerbated during the pill-free week. Unfortunately, if headaches are worsened on the pill, stopping the OC may not lead to immediate headache relief and improvement could take up to 12 months.

As with estrogen use, OC use in migraineurs is controversial due to the risk of stroke, particularly in association with the use of older, high dose pills. Recent studies suggest that while migraine is a risk factor for stroke, the increased risk is likely small in women who have migraine without aura and for women who do not have additional risk factors for stroke. Low dose, monophasic (not 'triphasic') OCPs are least likely to worsen migraine. If headaches worsen, different formulations may be tried and in some women, use of the OCP in a non-cycling fashion has had some success.

Pregnancy and the Postpartum

In some studies, 60-70% of women noted improvement in or alleviation of their migraine during pregnancy, particularly during the second or third trimesters. This improvement seemed more likely in women with migraine without aura and in women who previously experienced MM. Up to 10% of women may experience their first migraine attack during pregnancy. Thus, during pregnancy, a women's migraines may improve or worsen.

The greatest concern regarding treatment of migraine during pregnancy relates to the potential harm of drug therapy. Generally, migraine drugs should not be administered to pregnant patients or to women who are attempting to conceive. Reassurance, rest, ice packs and biofeedback (see Biofeedback - Chapter 4 - Alternatives) are often beneficial and may help the pregnant patient get through the first trimester, after which migraine may improve. For women who have severe migraine (often accompanied by nausea, vomiting and dehydration), medical therapy may be indicated, since this could pose a risk to the developing baby greater than the risk of medication itself. For severe attacks, intravenous fluids and an anti-nausea drug are often very beneficial. When migraine is frequent and disabling (3-4 prolonged, severe migraines per month), preventative therapy may be required.

Following delivery, migraine may reoccur, often by day 3-6 postpartum. If a woman chooses to breast feed, she should discuss this with her infant's pediatrician for the acceptable options for migraine pain relief.

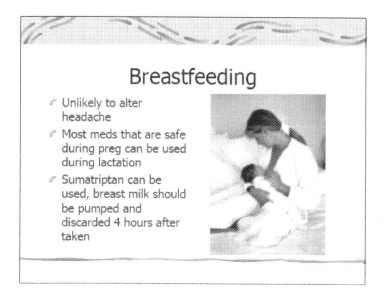

Medications considered 'safe' during pregnancy can also be used during breastfeeding, although the onset of headaches may be delayed during the breastfeeding stage.

Menopause

The changes in hormone levels occurring with menopause lead to a variable effect on migraine. Since estrogen production falls off, migraine may improve. However, hormone replacement therapy (HRT) often prescribed for symptoms of menopause, may worsen migraine. The type of menopause may also affect migraine such that two-thirds of women experiencing natural menopause tend to note improvement in migraine, while two-thirds of women undergoing surgical menopause tend to experience worsening of their migraine. Thus, hysterectomy is never recommended for treatment of menopausal migraine.

Management can be difficult for women who require hormone replacement therapy, but for whom such treatment worsens migraine: (1) reduce the dose of estrogen, (2) change the type of estrogen preparation (synthetic to natural or vice versa),

131

(3) employ continuous administration of cyclical (especially if headaches are associated with estrogen withdrawal) and (4) use of estrogens which provide more uniform levels - patch, vaginal estrogens. Given the recent results of the Women's Health Initiative and changes in recommendations against widespread HRT use, prescribing hormone/estrogen replacement therapy for migraine benefits alone, should be carefully thought out and used on a short-term basis only.

While the hormonal fluctuations can be a frustrating time for women who suffer with headaches, new insights into the pathophysiology effects of these hormones have provided us with a clearer picture and demonstrated the tremendous advancements in the understanding of migraine, leading to new therapeutic options. Following a logical step-by-step approach, with individualization of therapy tailored to the individual and perseverance on the part of both patient and doctor, usually leads to success.

Pregnancy & Headache
Patricia Mandalfino, M.D., F.R.C.P. C
Neurologist Interested in Headache
Kitchener, ON, Canada

Pregnancy and headache are common conditions and therefore co-occur frequently. Management of headache in the pregnant patient is a special situation since any diagnostic or therapeutic decision must take into account risk to the developing fetus.

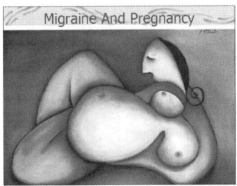

Migraine And Pregnancy

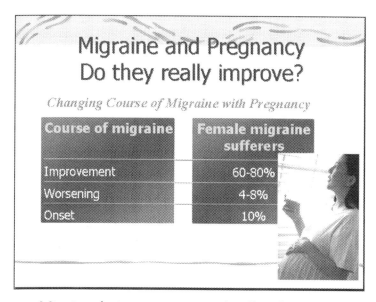

Migraine and Pregnancy
Do they really improve?

Changing Course of Migraine with Pregnancy

Course of migraine	Female migraine sufferers
Improvement	60-80%
Worsening	4-8%
Onset	10%

Migraines during pregnancy may be affected in one of three ways, although the 'trend' in most women is that of improvement.

It has been long established that hormonal fluctuations, particularly those of estrogen, impact migraine. Since pregnancy is a time of significant hormonal changes, changes in migraine patterns in pregnancy are common. Fortunately, pregnancy can be kind to many migraineurs. In particular, about two-thirds of women who suffer migraine without aura will have improvement in their headaches during the second and third trimesters associated with a rise in estrogen levels. This is particularly true for women sufferers whose headaches vary with their menstrual cycles. In contrast, women who have migraine with aura usually notice no change and sometimes there may even be worsening. Migraine sufferers, with and without aura, usually revert to their pre-pregnancy pattern following delivery and resumption of their menstrual cycles. Many migraine sufferers worry that their headaches pose risk to the developing fetus. This is not the case unless headaches are very severe and associated with protracted vomiting or inappropriate medication use.

The situation for tension type headaches is different. Tension type headaches are largely unaffected by hormone levels and therefore by pregnancy. Cluster headaches are infrequent in women of child-bearing age and therefore are not usually an issue in pregnancy.

It must be emphasized that any significant change in headache patterns or the new onset of headache in pregnancy or the post-partum period mandates evaluation by a physician. Pregnancy is a time of enormous physiologic changes which place individuals at higher risk for conditions that often present with headache. These include subarachnoid hemorrhage (bleeding in the brain), venous thrombosis (blood clots), certain tumors and pregnancy-induced hypertension (high blood pressure). Evaluation may require tests such as CT or MRI of the head. Particularly CT may pose risk to the fetus because of radiation (MRI risks are less well established). The physician should discuss the risks of any investigative procedure against the anticipated benefit and only proceed when benefit outweighs risk. Fortunately, a thorough history and physical examination often negates the need for tests. However, expert opinion holds that if CT scans or MRI are deemed necessary they should not be withheld because of the pregnancy.

Management of the Pregnant Headache Sufferer

In most instances, physician and pregnant patient are in agreement to avoid medication as much as possible. Non-pharmacological measures should be maximized before medication use is entertained. Massage, relaxation and biofeedback may be beneficial to many. Avoidance of triggers is critical. Patients should be encouraged to avoid any dietary triggers including alcohol and excess caffeine. Adequate sleep is essential since irregular sleep patterns are known as a migraine trigger. This may even include modifying work hours through the pregnancy. My personal experience is that employers are accommodating when medical documentation is provided. Your doctor should be an advocate in dealing with an employer. The "short-term pain" of lifestyle changes is viewed by the majority as a small price to pay for the "long-term gain" of ensuring the best fetal outcome.

Despite the best efforts, some patients may not be able to adequately control their headaches with non-pharmacological measures. A decision may then be able to proceed with medications and this should be done in conjunction with the obstetrician. Delaying medication until at least the second trimester and then only using the smallest dose for the shortest time are the goals. Non-pharmacological adjuncts described previously should be maintained as their benefits may minimize the need for medication. The list of "safe" medications in pregnancy is short but certainly adequate to control headaches in the vast majority of patients. I should emphasize that most over-the-counter and prescription medications should be avoided and therefore a physician should be consulted before any medication is used. This includes so-called "natural" remedies and vitamin supplements.

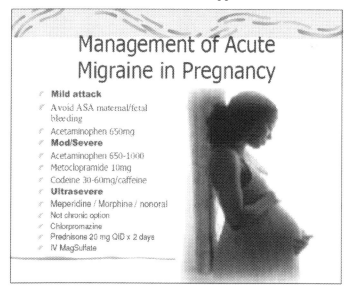

Management of Acute Migraine in Pregnancy

- **Mild attack**
- Avoid ASA maternal/fetal bleeding
- Acetaminophen 650mg
- **Mod/Severe**
- Acetaminophen 650-1000
- Metoclopramide 10mg
- Codeine 30-60mg/caffeine
- **Ultrasevere**
- Meperidine / Morphine / nonoral
- Not chronic option
- Chlorpromazine
- Prednisone 20 mg QID x 2 days
- IV MagSulfate

The 'do no harm' approach to migraine in pregnancy is always recommended, however when refractory headache and dehydration occur treatment should be considered.

As a final note, a difficult situation arises when women discover they are pregnant after they have used a variety of medications. Make certain to inform your doctor about any intention to become pregnant before treatment decisions are made.

Slides and comments are courtesy of Dr. Rose Giammarco, Hamilton Headache Clinic, Hamilton, Ontario, Canada

Summary

- Any new headache or change in pre- existing headaches in pregnancy should be evaluated by a physician.

- Migraine headaches are not usually a risk to the developing fetus unless ultra-severe (eg. with protracted vomiting).

- Non-pharmacological (non-drug) measures should be the mainstay of treatment wherever possible.

- Medications (including the over-the-counter, natural and prescribed) should only be used with physician supervision.

Menopause

Many women, after menopause, experience a discontinuation of their headaches. This is directly connected to the fact that their body stops producing estrogen, which we know has high influence on serotonin, the neurotransmitter that plays a key role in the onset of a headache. *(See Menopause in Migraine - online interview at www.headache-help.org - Q# 7)* (click on the interview graphic in the centre of our webpage at www.headache-help.org)

The good news for some migraine sufferers is that they can likely expect a discontinuation, or a reduction of their migraines after menopause. Unfortunately, for a small percentage of some migraine sufferers, menopause can actually "worsen" their headaches - but this is usually not the case.

Estrogen Replacement Therapy in Menopause

Often, women take female hormone pills at menopause and some possible symptoms experienced with menopause include; excessive or prolonged periods, osteoporosis, hot flashes, vaginal dryness, excessive sweating and depression. In some cases, the use of ERT (Estrogen Replacement Therapy, also called "Hormone Replacement Therapy") can actually worsen migraine headaches.

There are documented studies which show that sometimes women who choose estrogen replacement therapy, such as the estrogen patch, may actually experience worsening of their headaches as migraine sufferers.

The obvious benefits of HRT tend to far outway the potential problems associated with it and for this reason potential problems tend to be overlooked.

If headache sufferers insist on staying on the pill and continue to have headaches, NSAIDs (Nonsteroidal Anti-inflammatory Drugs) are generally recommended. Please consult with a physician or headache neurologist.

To learn more about the intricate relationship between hormones and headaches try to locate the book - *(Hormones & Headaches, by Dr. Seymour Diamond of the National Headache Foundation, Chicago, Illinois, USA or at a used bookstore as it is likely out of print). The National Headache Foundation website is www.headaches.org*

Susan Hutchinson, MD

Family Medicine, Women's Medical Group of Irvine, Irvine, CA. Migraine is very common in women during child-bearing years. Many women need or desire contraception, or may have other conditions such as endometriosis, severe dysmenorrhea, menorrhagia or acne for which may benefit from combination oral contraceptive treatment. Is it is safe to let women migraine

137

patients take oral contraceptives? What are the risks? Are there certain dosages or formulations that may be better than others for women with migraine?

The most commonly used forms of oral contraceptives (OC) are a combination of ethinyl estradiol and a progestin. These are often referred to as 'combination hormonal contraception' or 'combination oral contraceptives'. Less commonly used is the progestin-only containing OC, often referred to as the "mini-pill". OCs differ from hormone replacement therapy in several ways.

They work by blocking ovulation and changing the cervical mucus and the lining of the uterus. Hormonal replacement therapy, as is commonly used in menopause, contains a much lower dose of estrogen/progesterone that is not sufficient to block ovulation and prevent pregnancy.

SHOULD ORAL CONTRACEPTIVES BE USED TO TREAT MIGRAINE?

The use of oral contraceptives to prevent migraine is not clearly supported in studies or in the medical literature. Non-hormonal preventive agents such as the antiepileptic drugs, beta-blockers and antidepressants should be the mainstay of treatment in women needing a daily preventive. However, for those women, who need or want contraception, then using a monophasic low-dose combination contraceptive in a continuous fashion would theoretically help the migraine condition by keeping estradiol levels steady. This could be especially helpful for women suffering from menstrual migraines.

MIGRAINE, ORAL CONTRACEPTION, AND THE RISK OF STROKE

The type of migraine is important when considering the risk of stroke. Women with migraine without aura have a low risk of stroke and venous thromboembolism (VTE), similar to women without migraine.

Combination OC use increases a woman's risk for VTE and ischemic stroke. Observational studies found 1-3 additional cases of VTE among 10,000 women taking combination contraceptives for one year [1].

Taking into account a baseline 10-year ischemic stroke rate of 2.7 per 10,000 young women (ages 25-29) years, OC usage increases the risk to 4.0. The risk increases to 11.0 for women who have migraine with aura, and to 23.0 for women with migraine with aura using OC [2].

The World Health Organization (WHO) recommends that women with migraine with aura avoid combination contraceptive use [3].

The American College of Obstetricians and Gynecologists (ACOG) recommends using alternative forms of contraception in certain populations of women such as women over 35 years who smoke and women with migraine headaches [4].

There is little indication that OCs have a clinically important effect on headache activity in most women. Headache that occurs during early cycles of OC use tends to improve or disappear with continued use. No evidence supports the common clinical practice of switching OCs to treat headache. [5]

Combination OC are not recommended for some women with migraine. The screening history on such patients includes the following questions:
1. Is there a clotting disorder or history of deep venous thrombosis?
2. Are there risk factors for deep venous thrombosis or stroke? Take into account family history of heart attack or stroke under age 60 and cardiovascular risk factors such as age, high blood pressure, high cholesterol, low HDL cholesterol, obesity, smoking and high-sensitivity CRP (Reynolds Risk Score: Calculating Heart and Stroke Risk for Women)[6].
3. Does the patient experience migraine aura symptoms?

SPECIFIC ORAL CONTRACEPTIVE FORMULATIONS

Oral contraceptive pills come in two types of formulations. In monophasic oral contraception, all the "active" pills contain the same amount of ethinyl estradiol and progestin (traditional pack: 21 days active/7 days placebo). The 'active' pills in triphasic formulations vary in the amount of ethinyl estradiol and/or the progestin (traditional pack: 21 days active/7 days placebo). Some newer formulations of extended monophasic forumulations include cycles of 84 active pills/7 days placebo or 24 active pills/4 days placebo.

RECOMMENDATION FOR MIGRAINE PATIENTS

A low-dose (35 mcg ethinyl estradiol or less) monophasic OC may be used in most women with migraine. There are no good data to suggest that the lower dose formulations of 20-30 mcg ethinyl estradiol are any safer than the 35 mcg when looking at VTE or ischemic stroke risk. Using the OC in a continuous-dose regimen (skipping the placebo pills) may theoretically help prevent menstrual migraine. One study showed an incidence of headaches of 9.7% in women using extended-regimen OC vs. 17.3% in those using standard regimen OC. Any monophasic oral contraceptive can be adapted to be used in a continuous (extended) fashion.

FINAL COMMENTS

OC are not contraindicated for most women with migraine headaches. Once these women are successfully screened and start taking an OC, appropriate follow-up to monitor the headache pattern is crucial. The patient must be counseled to report new onset aura symptoms or changes in cardiovascular risk status should be reported to the health care provider. The OC should be discontinued if migraines worsen after the first few months of treatment or if the patient develops aura. Close collaboration among all treating health care providers is essential in caring for this large population of women migraine patients who need or want oral contraception.

REFERENCES

1. Gomes MP, Deitcher SR. Risk of venous thromboembolic disease associated with hormonal contraceptives and hormonal replacement therapy: a clinical review. Arch Intern Med 2004;164:1965-76.

2. Becker WJ. Use of oral contraceptives in patients with migraine. Neurology 1999;53 (4 suppl 1):S19-25.

3. World Heath Organization. Improving access to quality care in family planning. 3rd ed. Geneva, Switzerland: Reproductive Health and Research, World Health Organization, 2004.

4. ACOG Committee on Practice Bulletins-Gynecology. ACOG Practice Bulletin. The use of hormonal contraception in women with coexisting medical conditions. Number 18, July 2000. Int J Gynaecol Obstet 2001;75:93-106.

5. Loder E. et al. Headache as a side effect of combination estrogen-progestin oral contraceptives: a systematic review. Am J Ob Gyn. 2005;193:636-649

6. www.reynoldsriskscore.org

Reprinted with permission from:
Dr. Lawrence Robbins
Headache Neurologist
Robbins Headache Clinic
Northbrook, Illinois

11

Headaches in Children, Adolescents & People Over 50

Why do Older Adults Sometimes Stop Getting Headaches?

Headaches in Children

The Migraine Trust's Migraine: a guide for young sufferers – a resource pack

The best way of managing migraine is to stop attacks from happening. The aim is to cut down the number of attacks and the pain that goes with them. Your child will probably need acute migraine treatment as well, as not all attacks will be avoided.

Migraine can be an unpredictable condition. Parent and children learn from experience that certain things can trigger an attack, but the influence of these triggers is complicated. It is possible that on one occasion a trigger will appear to bring on a migraine, but on another occasion it will have no effect. These confusing signs can happen because a combination of factors may be necessary to trigger an attack. Moreover, it is possible that a migraine may only be triggered when the brain is in a sensitive state. Research is ongoing to try to find out exactly what causes the sensitivity of the brain in migraine sufferers.

Children carry out a wide range of activities in a number of different environments, and are under many different pressures every day. It is possible, by making some changes to set up a regular routine, that you can make the attacks happen less often.

Sleep

Some children are particularly likely to get migraines if their sleep pattern is disturbed. This can include having too much sleep, as well as not having enough. Setting regular times for getting up and going to bed may help to avoid a migraine.

Dehydration

Dehydration is a key cause of migraine, especially in children who are very active. Following a routine of drinking regularly may mean asking permission from school to let your child drink during class.

Diet

The start of a migraine attack may trigger a craving for a certain kind of food. This can make it difficult to decide if the food eaten before the attack caused the migraine, or if the attack was starting anyway. Of course, your child should avoid anything that regularly triggers a migraine attack, but banning certain things altogether may be more of a punishment than a help. Thinking about when, rather than what, your child is eating may have a greater effect on their migraines. Following a routine that includes regular meal times may help to reduce the number of attacks. Again, you may need to speak to your child's school about them eating outside of normal break times.

Stress

Children can feel under pressure from a range of different things. Stress can come from other children, from worrying about exams, and from family problems. Dealing with stress can be difficult, and you can help by knowing about these pressures. Your child may find it helps to talk about how they feel. A child can learn specific ways to relieve tension and stress.

Exercise

For some children, sudden physical exercise, such as running, can trigger a migraine attack. Setting up a routine of taking regular exercise, rather than overdoing it, may help to stop attacks. Making sure your child has enough to drink can also help to reduce this trigger.

Health

Many children find that they are more likely to get a migraine when they are not feeling well for another reason. For example, you might find that your child often gets a migraine when they are suffering from a cold or a stomach bug. Some girls regularly suffer migraine attacks at the start of their monthly period. If these things trigger a migraine in your child, remember that avoiding other trigger factors at these times can help to avoid an attack.

Identifying triggers

Parents and children often know about certain triggers that can lead to migraine. It is important to record as much information as possible about the headaches, so you can spot the triggers. These other triggers may not be obvious at first. This is especially true if you or your child already have strong ideas about what is causing their headaches.

Relaxation techniques

Some migraine sufferers use ways of relieving physical tension to avoid attacks. For example, massage and physical therapy are used to help muscle pain in the neck and shoulder. A common cause of such pain in children is a heavy school bag. A bag on wheels (or 'pull along' bag), or a spare set of textbooks to keep at home, can help reduce the weight they have to carry.

Biofeedback

The biofeedback technique has been used to reduce the number of attacks and the pain of migraine in some sufferers.

Biofeedback training teaches people to control certain body functions they do not normally think about controlling.

For example, a headache sufferer could learn to raise the temperature of a part of the body, say the hands. Redirecting blood to the hands reduces blood flow in the head, and the headache pain eases.

You need professional help to learn the skill of biofeedback. Children have used the skill successfully. Once a sufferer learns the technique, it can be practiced anywhere.

From: *Migraine: a guide for young sufferers.* Other topics in the series:
1. Migraine – the facts
2. Migraine – the figures
3. The effect of migraine – and ways to limit it
4. Diagnosing migraine in children – headache features
5. Diagnosing migraine in children – attack phases
6. Diagnosing migraine in children – more serious headaches and common misunderstandings
7. Diagnosing migraine in children – getting it right
8. Measuring the effect of migraine – and principles of managing migraine
9. Managing migraine in children – avoiding attacks
10. Managing migraine in children – preventive medication
11. Managing migraine in children – concerns about medication
12. Managing migraine in children – acute and rescue medication
13. The role of your child, and of supervising adults

The kit also has an easy-to-read book for children answering questions such as *"What's your headache like?"*, *"Why does your head hurt?"*, and *"What should I do when I get a migraine?"*

To request your own copy of *Migraine: a guide for young sufferers*, contact:
The Migraine Trust
2nd Floor
55-56 Russell Square
London WC1B 4HP
Tel: 020 7436 1336
Fax: 020 7436 2880
Email: info@migrainetrust.org
www.migrainetrust.org

Reprinted with permission from WHA Registered Charity No. 1080527. Company Limited by Guarantee, registered in England and Wales No.3464207

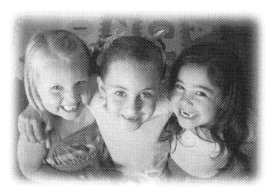

Adolescents & Headache
by Robert L. Hamel, Pa-C., Physician's Assistant, Michigan Headache & Neurological Institute, Ann Arbor, Michigan, USA

Adolescence is a difficult time. Adolescents experience multiple biological, social, psychological, and educational changes simultaneously. The addition of illness to this complex developmental process can be a small burden, or have a large impact, depending on individual circumstances. When the illness is head pain, pain management becomes dependent on a therapeutic alliance between the patient, parents, and healthcare professionals.

Who?

As boys get older, they tend to experience less migraine, a common type of adolescent headache. Perhaps due to the effects of estrogen, girls tend to experience more migraine.

Assessment

The history is the most important aspect of assessment. It is important to know whether a headache began suddenly and persisted, is intermittent associated with menstrual cycles, or has no apparent pattern. Headaches can evolve from intermittent to daily or become daily suddenly after a viral infection or injury. Distinguishing characteristics can emerge during this portion of the assessment, which helps to direct therapy.

Any change in headache, based on position of the body is important to note. Anatomical and fluid dynamic contributing factors to headache may be investigated based on a history of positional headache.

Other details are important to include the location of the headache, the character of the pain, associated symptoms (nausea, vomiting, light sensitivity, sound sensitivity, etc), what makes the pain worse, or what makes the pain better. In addition, pain does not occur in isolation. It is important to evaluate for mood as depression and anxiety may become aggravating influences if present before the pain, or may emerge as a result of the pain. Understanding the family's situation, i.e., divorce, separation, beginning a new school, and other socio-economic factors, may be important in assessing any developing impairment associated with head pain.

Unfortunately, some adolescents do use illicit substances. Specific questions directed at obtaining this information cannot be overlooked. This includes the use of tobacco and alcohol.

Relationships with peers in school may change as children become adolescents. Cruelty is common in school. School absence due to headache can become school avoidance if a child is "different", does not fit in, or is otherwise having difficulty progressing through a school culture. This can become a difficult problem to assess and requires the understanding and cooperation of professionals and parents with the goal of treating the head pain, but also expecting as much function as possible out of the individual adolescent.

Family medical history can shed light on parents' or grandparents' headaches or other pain disorders.

Physical examination is often normal in adolescents with headache. Indeed, the adolescent may appear to be not in pain at all, but reporting severe pain. This may be especially true of patients reporting daily pain. It is relatively easy to tell the difference between a girl with migraine headaches associated with menstrual cycles who is otherwise normal every other day of the month, versus a 16 year old who reports a severe daily headache. Both patients must be acknowledged as reporting what they feel. But in the case of the daily headache, a much more thorough investigation of all circumstances, medical, social, familial, and education would likely be important.

Physical examination should focus on areas of tenderness, neurological function, vital signs, and areas of sensitivity to light touch. In the case of daily headache it may be necessary to pursue a detailed laboratory investigation including cerebrospinal fluid analysis obtained after a lumbar puncture. MRI imaging of the brain and possibly the neck, and other laboratory tests.

Treatment

Treatment should be individualized. It may be as simple as providing a migraine abortive once or twice a month, or as complicated as providing medicine, psychological treatment, and interacting with school representatives and parents, and monthly medical visits.

Adolescents may be more responsive to cognitive behavioural techniques such as hypnosis, biofeedback, and relaxation techniques. Oral routes of medication are preferable to injectable or suppository use, whenever possible. Reliance on opiod medications should be avoided and early intervention by an experienced multidisciplinary pain management team whenever daily headache and significant school absence coexist is best.

In conclusion, adolescent headache can be a simple or extremely complicated problem, which, in either case, should be taken seriously by parents and medical professionals, as well as the adolescents themselves. Head pain is a condition that may evolve over time from intermittent to chronic, and early treatment to prevent rebound headache (medication overuse headache) and even disability status as an adult are good reasons for early intervention. Education becomes the focus of treatment in adolescents as migraine as other primary headache disorders are not susceptible to cure and often require a lifetime of treatment strategy.

Note: this article can be found at www.headache-help.org under the "free articles" button

Headaches and People Over 50
by Arthur Elkind, MD. Elkind Headache Center. Mount Vernon, NY
reprinted with permission from the American Council for Headache Education (ACHE) from the Newsletter of ACHE, Summer 1997, vol. 8, no. 2.

For many people, as we get older (and better) our headaches may improve too. Migraine headaches often become less severe and less frequent. The nausea, vomiting, light sensitivity and other symptoms may also lessen with age. Tension-type headache may continue unchanged if the individual has had it for much of his or her adult life.

Occasionally, the headaches may change in character or an older person who never had a significant problem before will suddenly develop headaches. When this occurs, it is important to have the headaches evaluated to rule out any underlying health problems.

Tension-type headache

It is not unusual for someone who had been largely headache-free to develop a chronic tension-type headache in their senior years. Often, this headache follows a major life change, such as retirement or a serious illness that has reduced mobility or independence. Someone who has just settled down to retirement may be puzzled and distressed at the onset of "tension" headache when all the pressure of the workplace is finally out of their lives.

On careful questioning, it often becomes clear that the headaches are related to an overall lowering of mood or a loss of enjoyment of life——to depression that may be slight or severe. Depression is only one of many possible causes of tension-type headache, but it should be suspected if the headaches follow some major change in situation. Retirement is often more stressful than many people expect, particularly if their work was important to their self-esteem. Treating the depression will generally relieve the headache.

A different kind of migraine

Older individuals will sometimes begin to have symptoms similar to a migraine aura (for example, weakness in the extremities, visual or sensory changes) with little or no headache. In many cases this turns out to be a peculiar form of migraine, called transient migraine accompaniments, that generally occurs after age 50. However, older persons who have these aura-like symptoms should not assume they are simply experiencing a different kind of migraine. The headaches should be carefully evaluated to rule out the possibility that the individual is experiencing episodes of a type of small, short-lasting stroke called transient ischemic attack (TIA).

A new study just published by Dr. Kathleen Merikangas offers the good news that migraine sufferers are not more prone to stroke as they grow older. On the contrary, the risk of stroke in a migraine sufferer is greater at 40 than at 70.

Headache as a symptom

As we get older, the chance that headache may be a symptom of some other problem becomes a greater concern. Whenever a patient reports a more severe or changed headache pattern, the doctor should do a careful history and examination to rule out the possibility that the headaches are related to some underlying disease.

Suspicion is greater if the elderly individual has other symptoms suggestive of illness, such as fatigue or unexplained weight loss. There is a condition called temporal arteritis or giant cell arteritis that occurs more often in older persons (over age 55), in which the larger arteries of the head become inflamed. Headache is often an early sign, with or without other symptoms such as joint pain, difficulty chewing, fever, blurred vision, weakness and weight loss. Typically, the headache is a continuous throbbing pain in the temples. If untreated, temporal arteritis can result in blindness and other serious complications. Fortunately, it responds well to treatment and is usually cured. Since early diagnosis is essential to preventing complications, you should see your doctor promptly if you develop throbbing temporal headaches accompanied by any of these other symptoms. Unexplained weakness or weight loss should always be brought to your physician's attention.

The possibility that your headaches might be related to underlying disease should not make you fearful of seeing the doctor and "learning the truth." On the contrary, you may discover that your headaches arise from something so simple as poorly fitting dentures, which put pressure on the teeth and gums that can translate into pain in the head and sinus region.

Headache as a side effect

Older individuals are more likely to taking drugs for other chronic disorders, and headache is a known side-effect of many medications. If you have reason to believe a needed medication may be linked to an increase in headache frequency, you should contact your doctor. A reduction in dosage or change to a related medication can be tried to see if the headaches respond. For example, some medicines for high blood pressure may cause increased headache as a side effect, but others are effective in controlling both blood pressure and chronic headache. Do not stop your medication or skip doses without consulting your doctor.

Headache management

It's important for the older individual who begins having chronic headaches or experiences a different kind of headache to see the doctor for a thorough evaluation. While a younger person with occasional headaches may do very well just taking over-the-counter pain relievers, this is not a good option for the older person. People often assume that drugs that are sold without a prescription are perfectly safe. However, older individuals in particular may be more prone to develop bleeding ulcers with overuse of aspirin-containing drugs, and many of the common anti-inflammatory drugs can make high blood pressure worse.

The doctor treating the older patient for headache must do a more careful history and physical examination than may be required in a healthy young person. It is necessary to rule out any disease that may be related to the headache, such as temporal arteritis. Also, any other medical conditions that would limit the choice of headache medication, such as diabetes, chronic lung disease, glaucoma or enlarged prostate, need to be identified.

Individuals in the elderly age group will differ greatly in their ability to tolerate drugs at doses normally used in young or middle-aged adults. A 60-year-old may not be much different from a 40-year-old, but an 80-year-old will need to be treated more cautiously, starting with minimal doses and going up slowly. Liver and kidney function slow down with age, so that a drug is not processed and eliminated from the body quite as quickly. Too much of the drug may accumulate in the bloodstream, resulting in more severe side effects. This is a risk with the common over-the-counter pain medicines as well as prescription drugs.

Many headache medicines can be safely used even in the very old. Acetaminophen (Tylenol, Excedrin, and many prescription drugs) is generally safe for occasional use, and some older migraine sufferers can take sumatriptan (Imitrex) or an ergot drug (Cafergot, Wigraine, Bellergal or DHE) 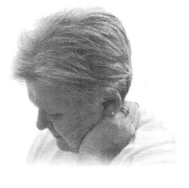 without excessive side effects. When a daily medication is needed to prevent frequent headaches, often it's possible to choose one that has other important benefits, such as controlling blood pressure.

Even more than younger age groups, the elderly may find that complaints of chronic headache are not taken seriously by those around them. There are effective treatments for all ages, and older persons who suffer from headache should find a sympathetic and knowledgeable doctor to help them.

12

Travel, Stress
and the Environment

*I am convinced my bad headaches are linked
to the environment.*

Travel and Headache
By R. Steven Singer, MD

We are about to begin the glorious season of the year when we wait in mile-long lines at Disneyland, have picnics with the ants, get sunburns because we forget to take along that lotion with the higher numbers after the name, and . . . have a good chance of more headaches.

Summer headaches may occur because of all those special traditions that associate with the season. First of all, we are likely to travel. Occasionally, just going up in altitude may trigger a headache. Most people who climb our local Mt. Rainier at 14,408 feet get some degree of headache, along with other symptoms. Any significant problem is unlikely below 8,000 feet, according to the traditional literature on "acute mountain sickness."

Admittedly, most of us are not going trekking in Nepal this July, nor are we climbing Mt. Rainier! We are, however, likely to fly somewhere, and that is also likely to trigger a headache. The barometric pressure change in airplane cabins is equivalent to altitudes of 3,600 to 6,500 feet, depending on the altitude of the plane and the type of aircraft. That appears sufficient to cause a severe throbbing migraine in some individuals, just like a change in the weather can in some people, with even less barometric pressure change.

Early last year, Dr. Richard Lipton wrote "Fair winds and foul headaches," a fascinating editorial in the journal Neurology on the subject of triggers. This paper commented on the interesting issue of weather and other triggers. There is no good explanation for barometric headache (or what one of my patients refers to as her "meteorological migraine"). Most of my patients who have "weather headaches" try to blame their sinuses, which is one factor that probably isn't responsible for all the pain and suffering. It is more likely that the lower oxygen level in the blood has something to do with it, but nobody knows. As Dr. Lipton notes in his article, quoting Canadian researchers Dr. Cooke and colleagues, look out for those warm Chinook winds up in Alberta, Canada. They can wreck your whole vacation if your headache is long enough and your vacation short enough.

The treatment of the lesser examples of high altitude headache (in the airplane) is the same as any other variety of migraine. A triptan, Midrin or DHE nasal spray would be fine. High altitude mountain sickness is an entirely different thing, but should be treated by descending to a lower attitude in a hurry, if possible. Other features of travel that may induce headache include sleep deprivation, jet lag, major dietary changes, general commotion, and stress. On the other side of the vacation equation, the positive side, are reduced stress, more sleep, and general "fun in the sun." One patient will tell us "I didn't have a single headache my whole vacation" and the next one will say "I had a headache every day." Most know which category they fit before they leave for their trip.

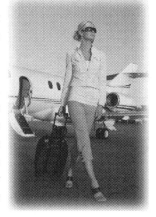

What can you do about "travel headache"? There is no simple solution, but being very aware of the triggers and avoiding the worst ones is important, even if that glass of free champagne on the plane looks very tempting. *"I also advise my patients to*

156

take twice as much of your usual medications with you as you would normally require, specifically the acute medications such as the triptans and nausea medications." Patients have told us stories of migraines occurring in strange and faraway places on this planet, and all the problems they encountered trying to get treatment--something that wouldn't have happened if they'd had been better prepared for the crisis.

It's important to remember that luggage can be lost or stolen on trips. It is preferable to have the medications on your person or in two places. If traveling overseas, there may be special restrictions on carrying medications, particularly narcotics. In general, if they're in the original prescription containers it isn't an issue. Some travel resources advise having the doctor write a brief note about the medications needed and the diagnoses. (Getting notes from doctors may not be that easy anymore, unfortunately.) Find out, in advance, if any of the countries being visited have specific regulations in this area.

There are other headache hazards in the summer months. The most cruel of all must certainly be the "ice cream headache." These headaches are often brief, very severe attacks of pain in the forehead or around the eye. They are likely to occur with the application of any type of extremely cold substance on the roof of the mouth or the throat. They are also much more likely to occur in people with migraine. Myself, I have the pleasure of these headaches with any kind of drink, including crushed ice. The origin of the pain is unclear but may be excessive blood vessel spasm (reflexive vasospasm) induced by the cold. I find it very easy to fix this kind of headache. Don't sit there with the offending agent in your mouth up against the hard palate for extended periods of time, even if it is the best strawberry Margarita you ever had.

Another cruel summer joke is the "hot dog headache," resulting from the nitrites in hot dogs and other cured meat products. The nitrites are believed to produce headache by causing dilation or expansion of the cranial vessels, which are pain sensitive. Looking at the last two topics, ice cream and hot dogs, we begin to see the problem of picnics, which include sun, hot dogs, some form of alcohol (beer?), cold beverages of other types, perhaps ice cream, and, if you're really unlucky, being hit on the head by a baseball at the company picnic.

Summer sun can induce a headache, particularly with long exposure. In a study reported in Headache last January, migraine patients were found to be more light sensitive than other people when headache-free as well as during their migraines. Some of these patients tell us that bright light or glare can bring on their migraine. It isn't necessary to advise them to use sunglasses. They learned that a long time ago. Patients with classical migraine, particularly with an aura involving visual disturbance, may be especially sensitive to visual triggers. I've seen two patients now who informed us that their migraine could be triggered by a light stimulus very similar to their usual visual aura. In other words, external mimics of their visual aura would commence a migraine. One man described being on his cabin cruiser looking out over the water, with the sun glimmering brightly off the waves. When he went down below decks, the same glimmering in vision continued in the relative darkness there, which was very much like his usual aura. His usual painful migraine followed. What can the boater do about that? Alas, don't forget your migraine medication and watch the other triggers.

I am left with two other summer headache concerns: motion sickness that you may encounter out there on your cabin cruiser and the infamous hangover that may follow your wine-tasting party in August.

Motion sickness must be mentioned because it is common among people with migraine, particularly in childhood. Sixty percent of adults with migraine report severe motion sickness during childhood. It often continues into adulthood and may occur with or without headache. Attacks may be triggered by odor, and, for women, are more likely to occur with the monthly period.

There is no good explanation for the common coexistence of these two disorders. A variety of medications can be used to treat motion sickness, such as promethazine, meclizine, or nausea medications. Aboard cruise liners, a shot of promethazine (Phenergan) is often supplied. Scopolamine patches have been used as well.

Hangover is a topic worthy of a short book. I felt it belonged here because summer seems to be very good time to have a party. For migraine sufferers, relatively modest amounts of alcohol may be sufficient to bring on a hangover, so don't try to keep up with Uncle Frank. The headache component appears to be triggered by a variety of organic chemicals including ethyl alcohol, aldehydes, methanol, formaldehyde and formic acid. Certain types of beverages are much more likely to cause hangover than others, starting at the top of the "bad list" with champagne, red wines, dark beers, followed by white wine, lighter beers, and lastly less complex substances like gin and vodka.

Our patients report that migraine drugs such as Midrin are often very effective for the headache of the hangover. Beyond that, we hope we won't be accused of preaching if we recommended that people not drink in amounts sufficient to produce a hangover in the first place.

Good luck this summer, all you migraine sufferers. We will just hope that all the good things about summer will outweigh the bad and reduce your probability of a day in your bed with the shades drawn and your pill bottles on your bedside table.
--R. Steven Singer, MD. NorthWest Headache Clinic. Kirkland, WA

Summertime Travel Tips
- Have headache medications easily accessible in a carry-on or tote bag.
- On trips, take twice as much of your headache medications with you as you would normally expect to need.
- Pack your headache medications in two separate places, in case any of your luggage is lost or stolen.

- To avoid problems with customs, keep your medications in their original prescription containers when traveling abroad.
- Take special care to avoid triggers such as alcohol, skipped meals or irregular sleep.

Reprinted with permission from the American Council for Headache Education (ACHE) from Headache, the Newsletter of ACHE, Summer 2001, vol. 12, no. 2.

Stress & Headache

Reprinted with permission from Alvin E. Lake, III, Ph.D. Michigan Headache & Neurological Institute, Ann Arbor, Michigan, USA

Most headache sufferers encounter many headache "experts" among their friends, acquaintances, work colleagues, and sometimes even their family members who tell them that their headaches are the result of either too much stress in their lives , or a failure to adequately deal with stress when you're too stressed - learn to relax. This kind of advice can be very irritating and sometimes do more harm than benefit, despite what may be the good intentions of the advice-giver. The sufferer feels blamed for the headache and misunderstood. What are the facts about stress and headaches as revealed by recent research?

Stress as a Headache Trigger/Aggravator

A recent study of 366 migraine patients who kept daily diaries for 3 months, documenting life events and headaches indicated that stress was identified as a factor preceding migraines for 42% of the patients. For comparison, the most prevalent trigger or aggravator was sleep disturbance/fatigue (80%). Food and drink sensitivities were identified by 36%. 35% identified weather changes as a trigger, and 32% women noted menstrual correlation. A separate study followed 100 consecutive children and adolescents with headache who were seen in primary care medical practices. "Tension" was identified as "always a trigger or aggravator" by 68%, and was more prevalent than other common migraine triggers such as bright lights (51%), loud noises (40%), and missed meals (29%).

Long-term diary studies of small groups of patients have found that there is a relationship between stress and headache. The most common finding is correlation between stress occurring on the day of the headache, often preceding it by a few hours. However, for some patients there is a significant correlation between a feeling of stress occurring 2 or 3 days before a migraine. However, these studies do not distinguish between feeling stressed due to life events, and the feeling that may be part of migraine prodrome - chemical changes in the brain that are actually part of developing a migraine. Prodromes do not trigger headaches. They represent a period of vulnerability that can result in a migraine unless protective action is taken.

The finding that stress may trigger or aggravate a headache does not indicate that stress is the cause of the headache. Migraine is a genetically-based, biological disorder. Once migraines emerge as a problem, then stress can be one of a number of risk factors that can combine to trigger an attack.

What is stress?

Technically, stress is a psychological response in the body, and the stressors are the events that trigger a stress response. Sometimes stress responses develop spontaneously, without the need for outside triggers. At a vulnerable time, minor life hassles may trigger a stress response. At less vulnerable times, the same event may be no more than a minor irritant. In fact, research has shown that it is the frequency of minor hassles that appears to have the greatest impact on migraine, while patients may rise to the occasion and effectively cope with a severe stressor (such as a heart attack in a spouse) while maintaining good headache control.

It is often the let down after a stressful period that triggers a headache. Examples include the end of a stressful work week, or the aftermath of a family illness. One of our patients who is a school teacher noted that her headaches often increased in frequency and severity during the summer, when the school period was over.

Her solution was to increase her involvement in outside activities during the summer, such as teaching summer school, which for her actually resulted in less headache activity.

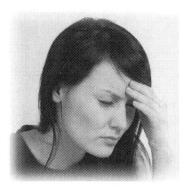

The headache itself is perhaps the most common and difficult stressor that confronts all headache sufferers. **Anxiety about possible or impeding headache, including fear of the inability to function, is certainly understandable.** Unfortunately, headache-related fear (cephalagiaphobia) can further increase headache vulnerability, aggravate a developing headache, or lead to over-use of analgesic or abortive medications.

What can be done about it?

1) Remain open to the possibility that stress could be a factor in your headaches. Try not to be defensive about it. Stress responses are normal, we all have them, and it is only in headache vulnerable individuals that may trigger a headache. Sometimes stress responses occur in situations where we least expect them. Try to take an attitude of "that's interesting" when you note a stress response. Make an effort to avoid self criticism. It is only when we recognize the presence of a stress response that we can do anything about it.

2) If people annoy you by harping on the stress connection, you can tell them "I know you are trying to help, I appreciate your concern, but please stop bringing this up. It is not helpful". You can take steps to educate people who are close to you, and really

want to learn more about headaches. With acquaintances, on the other hand, you may want to develop a thick skin and let some of their less helpful comments about your headaches roll off your back.

3) Close friends and family members can sometimes alert you to behavioural changes in yourself that may signal a stress response. Whether this is helpful or not depends on your relationship with that person, their willingness to do this in a truly compassionate way, and the extent to which you can be non-defensive about it.

4) Learn simple relaxation techniques. One simple but effective technique is to breathe from your abdomen (not your chest), and to slow your breathing down. For example, breathing in for 4 seconds and out for 4 seconds (4x4 breathing) can be a rapid and very effective method of calming yourself.

5) Be proactive, not reactive. The best time to manage stress is before you feel stressed. Many stressors are predictable. If you know that you will be confronting a difficult situation, then relax before it happens. Once a stress response becomes full-blown, it is much more difficult to relax- the chemical changes have to run their course.

6) Manage stressful behaviour. Our actions can create stress, such as when a headache sufferer tries to get as much done as possible when they think a headache may be coming on. Slow down. Get adequate sleep (remember, sleep disturbance is the most prevalent migraine trigger!) Eat regular meals. Take breaks. Give yourself enough time to get things done, and set realistic goals.

7) Manage your worries - our thoughts and negative anticipations of events can be just as distressing as the events themselves. Sometimes the anticipation of a stressful event is worse than the event itself. Try catching a stream of negative thoughts early, and ask yourself "is this type of thinking going to hurt me or help me?" Practice thought-stopping - tell yourself "stop!" and then

distract yourself with some other activity to get negative thinking off your mind. This takes practice and consistency, but can be very helpful.

8) Work on reducing your fear of pain. Self-talk can help - "One step at a time. You can handle this."

9) Do not be afraid to seek psychological help. Even a few sessions of professional help in learning biofeedback and stress-management techniques, and talking over your reactions to the stressors in your life, can assist you in further developing your headache-coping skills. We are social beings, and the ability to seek and accept help from others is a strength, not a weakness.

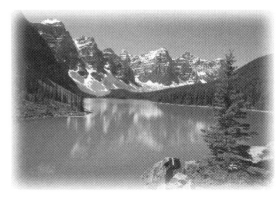

Environment and Headache

In Canada, many of the 3.4 million migraine sufferers are often triggered by foods, weather changes, stress, changes in sleep patterns, and hormonal fluctuations in women. (2007, Merck Frosst Canada)

So why is it so important for a migraine sufferer to learn their triggers? So that they can avoid triggering headaches unnecessarily. Migraine triggers are helpful in physicians diagnosing migraine.

Weather changes can be further broken down as barometric pressures (altitude), bright sunlight, and in western Canada - the

Chinook winds. Storm fronts can also be an aggravating factor. Atmospheric pressure has also been recorded by some migraine sufferers as an environmental trigger that can bring on a migraine attack.

It has often been recorded that barometric pressure fluctuations can bring on a migraine. See Travel and Headache - Chapter 12.

Significant weather changes include sunshine, thunderstorms, and changing atmospheric pressure. Many migraine sufferers also complain about the bright lights that are reflected from the snow in winter.

The spring season has more frequent migraine headache attacks, and there is a slightly higher occurrence in female migraine sufferers, over male.

Many unfortunate migraine sufferers are commonly triggered by weather changes as well as other factors. Regrettably, little is known about the relationship between environment and headache.

Sufferers sometimes can drift from doctor to doctor, at times clog emergency rooms, sometimes seek out alternative methods that are not tested, and occasionally become alienated from the medical profession.

One study reported that 50% of migraine sufferers reported that weather was a significant trigger for their migraine headaches.

Many studies are controversial, but most agree that weather plays a major trigger-factor for many migraine sufferers.

In closing, if headache sufferers and their physicians play close attention to weather-triggers - and how they apply to that migraine sufferer's headache pattern - it is very possible to be ready with acute migraine medication, when the next environmentally-induced migraine headache attack occurs. Weather triggers are difficult to avoid, but if significant weather changes are imminent, the migraine sufferer can take care to avoid other avoidable headache triggers which might add up with the weather trigger to bring on a migraine.

By Brent Lucas, Headache Researcher, Help for Headaches, London, Canada

Reviewed by Dr. Werner J. Becker, MD, FRCPC (neurol)
Professor, Dept of Clinical Neurosciences
Faculty of Medicine
University of Calgary
Calgary, Alberta, Canada.

1. The effect of Weather on Headache
Patricia B. Prince, MD; Alan M. Rapoport, MD; Fred D. Sheftell, MD; Stewart J. Tepper, MD; Marcelo E. Bigal, MD, PhD

2. *Effect on the Chinook Winds on the probability of migraine headache occurrence.*
J. Piorecky; W. J. Becker, MD; M.S. Rose, PhD

3. *Precipitating Factors in Migraine: A Retrospectrive Review of 394 Patients*
Lawrence Robbins, MD. Assistant. Professor., Rush Medical College, University of Illinois, Robbins Headache Clinic

4. Cooke LJ, Rose MJ, Becker WJ, Chinook winds and migraine headache, *Neurology 2000: 54: 302-7*

13

How to Prepare for Your Physician's Appointment, Record keeping and Persons with a Disability

Come to your physician's appointment prepared!

How to Prepare for your Physician's Appointment

Doctor's diagnose headaches according to a list of symptoms as set out by the classification committee of the International Headache Society in 1998. So it is with little surprise that physicians and researchers are always pushing headache sufferers to learn their symptoms. Learning these features or symptoms can save you time, money and increase your quality of life.

When a person becomes diabetic the first thing he or she does is to work with a diabetic nurse to find out which type of diabetes they may have, in order to begin proposed treatments as recommended for that particular type. Treating headache or migraine should be approached in the same manner.

Listed below is an article called "How Doctors Diagnose Headache"

How Doctors Diagnose Headache
By Donald J. Dalessio, MD., Scripps Clinic and Research Foundation, La Jolla, California

Every year, nearly three-quarters of the population have headaches. Of all the visits to physician's and emergency rooms, a little over 1% are for headache. Sufferers from severe headache sometimes fear they must have a brain tumour or hemorrhage. However, benign headaches can be just as intensely painful as those resulting from a malignant disease. Although tumour, abscess, hemorrhage and meningitis only rarely cause chronic headache, the first concern is to rule out these possibilities. A physical exam, neurological evaluation and a variety of tests are used to detect any underlying cause, such as hypertension (high blood pressure) or fever and infection. Chronic headaches are seldom due to sinus or dental problems, or to infection or allergies.

There are no precise clinical tests that serve to make the diagnosis of migraine, tension-type, cluster, or other benign headache condition. Instead, the physician depends greatly on the headache sufferer's accuracy in describing the symptoms, the pattern of the headaches, and any suspected triggers.

How long have you had these headaches?

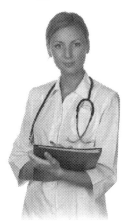

Migraine will lessen at menopause, but it will sometimes begin at that time. If a patient takes estrogen during the menopausal period, it will often prolong the estrogen influence well beyond menopause. Tension-type headaches can begin at any time of life.

Do other members of your family get headaches?

Migraine runs in families, but cluster headache usually does not. Cluster headache is more common in men than women, while migraine is much more common for women.

How often do you get these headaches?

Your doctor will ask you to estimate how many headaches you get per year. This will be important in deciding whether the treatment approach should be prophylactic (preventing the headaches) or abortive (stopping a headache attack in progress).

If headaches are recorded on a "per week/per month/per year basis", headaches that are more frequent can be better identified.

Has the pattern or frequency changed?

People often seek medical attention because headaches have become more severe or more frequent. For example, a person who has occasional severe headaches might develop a secondary pattern of milder daily headaches. In this case it's necessary to diagnose the primary headache condition and then try to discover the factors that might be making the headaches worse.

Where in the head do you feel the pain?

Pain that is on one side of the head and sometimes changes sides during the attack suggests the possibility of migraine. Migraine pain can occur anywhere in the head or face but most often in the temple. Severe pain in and around the eye and temple can be characteristic of a cluster headache, if other symptoms are present. Tension-type headache can be on one or both sides of the head.

> "Pain that is on one side of the head and sometimes changes sides during the attack suggests the possibility of migraine."

The pain may be in the front of the head but it is often most severe in the neck, shoulders and back of the head. Severe pain in and around there can be a cluster headache, if other symptoms are also present. Cluster headaches are generally confined to one side of the head, usually to the eye.

Describe the pain for me?

Migraine pain is typically throbbing or pulsating. A dull, nagging, persistent pain is more characteristic of tension-type headache. This pain is sometimes described as tight and constricting or as a feeling of pressure. The pain of cluster headache is deep and penetrating, as though a hot poker were driven into the eye.

For symptoms of a chronic daily headache please refer to chapter 9 - "Is this a chronic daily headache?"

What other symptoms do you have with the headache attack?

Loss of appetite, nausea and vomiting occur most commonly with migraine, and these are sometimes more incapacitating than the headache itself. Neck stiffness or tenderness often occurs with tension-type headache, but can also occur with migraine, often at the beginning of the migraine attack, and can of course occur where there are problems with the back of the head or neck. Sufferers of both migraine and tension-type headache tend to have a habit of grinding or clenching their teeth, and some people with jaw problems can actually incite a migraine by eating, chewing or grinding.

> "...and some people with jaw problems can actually incite a migraine by eating, chewing or grinding"

Redness or tearing of the eye and nasal congestion on the side with the headache are symptoms of cluster headache. Light and sound sensitivity during the attack are very common for migraine sufferers.

How long does the headache attack last?

Migraine by definition of the International Headache Society lasts from 4 hours to 72 hours. The aura associated with migraine with aura can last up to 20 minutes. Generally, a migraine sufferer has headache-free periods between attacks. Tension-type headache and chronic migraine can persist for days or continually. Cluster headache by definition goes from approximately 30 to 45 minutes to 128 minutes.

Often migraine headaches co-exist with Chronic Daily Headaches. It is advisable to consult with a skilled physician with a keen interest in headaches.

Diaries and Record Keeping

Keeping a diary and communicating those features to your physician is very important. There are many kinds of headaches and each have their associated symptoms which allows your doctor to make a diagnosis so that a treatment plan can begin.

Below I have listed some of the "typical" questions that a physician may ask you. Coming prepared to your appointment can take some of the guesswork out of "diagnosing your particular headache" and sent a positive message to your physician that you are willing to help yourself. Physicians are very busy and coming prepared to your appointment makes good sense.

I, myself, like the concept of being a "proactive patient" which also enables me to be part of the "problem-solving" phase.

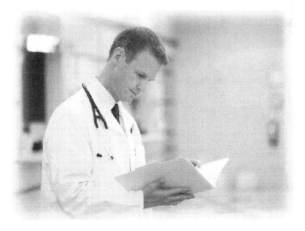

How long have you suffered from these headaches? Does anyone else in your family suffer?

What makes your headaches better? What makes them worse? (Eg. Bending over)

What location of your head are your headaches at? Do they move over time?

How would you describe your headaches? (Eg. Pounding, squeezing, drilling, dull aching, constant aching, stabbing)

Are your headaches predictable? (Eg. Storm fronts, travel, seasons, high altitudes, sun exposure)

What changes have occurred in frequency, quality, or symptoms from the beginning of your headache years until now? (in other words 'how has your headache pattern changed'?)

Do certain foods seem to trigger or induce a headache? (Eg. coffee, aged cheese, red wine, MSG - monosodium glutamate), citrus fruits. (refer to chapter 7 - Headache Triggers) Do certain physical exercises make them worse? Do bright lights or strong odours bring them on?

How long do the headaches last? Does the headache seem to take a holiday?

What method of treatment seems to help? Make a list of all treatments tried before that are ineffective? Did you give them long enough to work?

Do you have any warning signs such as tingling sensations, faster heart rate, numbness, dizziness, short-temperedness or irritability, before the headache?

For women only:
Menstruation and Menopause
Are your headaches associated with your menstrual period? Do they disappear at menopause? See Chapter 10 - Hormones

& Women With Headache? **Does ERT (Estrogen Replacement Therapy or the "pill") make the headaches worse?**

<u>Pregnancy</u>
Do your headaches change during pregnancy? Do they go away or did they get worse, or unaffected? Do they get worse after delivery or after breast feeding?

On a scale of 1-10, with 1 being the least and 10 being the worst - can you rate your headaches? (Upon waking, mid-day, evening)

Are your headaches better if you seek out a nice quiet dark room? Are they worse with activity? (Eg. Exercise, orgasm) If your headaches are related to sexual intercourse there is a headache condition called *coital headache* **that you may wish to search for on the internet.**

We know that sleep disturbances and headache are highly linked. Do you have difficulty falling asleep at night? Do you wake up with a headache in the morning? Do you wake up frequently throughout the night?

Are your headaches associated with stress, such as a stressful event? Are your headaches predictable after a stressful period is finished? (Eg. weekends, holidays) Do you get "let-down" headaches (after company has left)? Do holidays or something entertaining make them worse? (See Chapter 12 - Stress)

Are your headaches worsened by your Fibromyalgia (if you have it?) Headaches can also be a symptom of fibromyalgia. (Refer to Chapter 9 - Fibromyalgia and Headache)

Editors Note: The presence of one or more headaches will require careful record keeping and may make "identifying one headache category" very difficult. Most valid treatments exert an effectiveness in some, but not all patients, and finding the one or a few treatments that work for you will raise your quality of life. Good record keeping is a great way to "isolate" your headache type so treatment options can be discussed. Answering and responding to these questions can help you in the "sorting out" stage and can greatly reduce the guesswork, so that options to investigate are not as plentiful. Only your doctor is qualified to make a diagnosis. This fast checklist is not intended to replace a physician's advice, but to assist you in narrowing down the possibilities.

Reviewed and updated by Dr. Joel Saper, Michigan Headache & Neurological Institute, Ann Arbor, Michigan

Headaches and Persons with a Disability

Headache as a Disability
by Brent Lucas
Help for Headaches
London, Canada

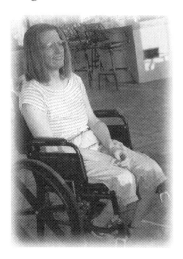

When we talk about headaches and disabilities, we need to differentiate between those who are disabled and get migraines and those who are disabled due to their severe headaches.

I will not go into the MIDAS (Migraine Disability Assessment Questionnaire) online test, as it is thoroughly covered in Chapter 8. (See Chapter 8 - Tests.)

Head pain can be cunning and elusive for some "headache experts" to properly diagnose and treat. Many times people show up at walk-in clinics or emergency rooms (see Chapter 8, Emergency Rooms) because they just cannot bear the internal, agonizing pain they feel, which has often led to disablement. When you think of a disability you quickly think of some unfortunate who is wheelchair bound, or someone who is bed-ridden - you certainly don't think of a headache as disabling. Many of us who are headache sufferers have had to alter work plans because the headache becomes unbearable.

Some **open legal issues** concerning headache as a disability, or workplace safety and insurance issues, do not, in most cases, reflect the treatment of many headache physicians. (Gallagher,1999). In most of the documented cases the treating physician wishes to remain uninvolved and avoids the issue - thereby placing the sufferer to "go it alone".

Being on a disability claim from work can mean higher health benefits and less productivity. So it is to the companies' financial gain to review claims even if these claims differ in their magnitude and complexity. But what about the person who cannot continue working due to their headache severity? Is there not a price tag for the day-to-day suffering the headache person endures? Is piece of mind only a luxury because of socio-economic factors, or because of access to a medical professional that will validate their claim?

Both temporary and permanent disabilities are something that unions rarely sink their teeth into. They generally refer claims to the health and safety representative who in turn, contacts an organization like ours (there are only a few headache groups in Canada). So you see, getting someone to advocate for you can be very hard, let alone produce substantial results for you or your spouse.

Being on a disability claim can mean ability, not disability. Volunteering with a charity like ours can mean a wealth of knowledge which can lead to future experiences. Knowing where to put your fingers on a certain "headache-related" issue, can really be helpful. A better understanding of your condition can put you back in the driver's seat - not locked out of your car without a coat hanger!

Editor's note:

For those persons with a disability that have hearing or sight limitations - there is an interview on the Help for Headaches homepage - www.headache-help.org - with a Neurologist in Canada. Click on the interview image at the centre-bottom of our charity website homepage. Each interview question is published with answers in text format (hard of hearing) and in audio format (blind persons). This program is brought to you by an unrestricted educational grant from Pfizer Pharmaceuticals Canada.

14

Drawing from Resources
to Help You Sort Out

Canada

Help for Headaches
515 Richmond Street
Box #1568, STN B
London, ON, Canada
N6A 5M3
Tel - 519.434.0008
brent@helpforheadaches.org
www.headache-help.org

World Headache Alliance
info@w-h-a.org
www.w-h-a.org

Headache Network Canada
www.headachenetwork.ca

Migraine Zero (Francais)
Contact: Jaime Lim, B.A., M.A - jaime.lim@mail.mcgill.ca

United States

American Council for Headache Education (ACHE)
19 Mantua Road
Mt. Royal, NJ
07061
Tel- 856.423.0258
Fax - 856.423.0082
achehq@talley.com
www.achenet.org

MAGNUM
113 South Saint Asaph Street
Suite #300
Alexandria, Virginia
22314
www.migraines.org

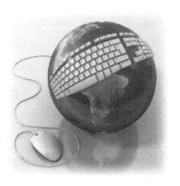

National Headache Foundation
820 N. Orleans
Suite 217
Chicago, Illinois
60610
Tel - 1.888.NHF.5552
info@headaches.org
www.headaches.org

Major US Headache Centres & Clinics

Michigan Headache & Neurological Institute
3120 Professional Drive
Ann Arbor, Michigan
48104-5131
Tel - 734.667.6000
Fax - 734.667.2422
www.mhni.com

Robbins Headache Clinic
1535 Lake Cook Road
Northbrook, Illinois
60062
Tel - 847.480.9399
Fax - 847.480.9044
www.headachedrugs.com

New York Headache Center
30 East 76th Street
New York, NY
10021
www.nyheadache.com

New England Center for Headache
30 Buxton Farm Road
Stamford, Connecticut
06905
Tel - 203.968.1799
Fax - 203.968.8303
je@nech.net
www.headachenech.com

Multidisciplinary Headache Clinic
Pain & Evaluation & Treatment Institute
Dawn A. Marcus, MD, FRCP(C)
5750 Center Avenue
Pittsburgh, PA 15206
University of Pittsburgh, PA
www.dawnmarcusmd.com

Oregon Headache Clinic
19001 SE McLaughlin Blvd.
Milwaukee, Oregon
97267
Tel - 503.656.9844
Fax - 503.656.3120
noheadaches@migrainesurvival.com
www.migrainesurvival.com

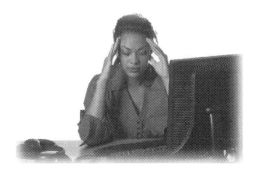

Europe

European Headache Federation
c/o Kenes International
17 rue du Cendrier
P.O. Box 1726
Switzerland
Tel - +41 22 906 9154
Fax - +41 22 732 2852
info@ehf-org.org
www.ehf-org.org

Migraine Trust
2nd Floor, 55-56 Russell Square
London
WCIB 4HP
Tel - 020.7436.1336
Fax - 020.7436.2880
info@migrainetrust.org
www.migrainetrust.org

Migraine Action Association
27 East Street
Leicester LE1 6NB
Tel – 0116 275 8317
Fax – 0116 254 2023
info@migraine.org.uk
www.migraine.org.uk

The City of London Migraine Clinic
22 Charterhouse Square
London, England
EC1M 6DX
Tel - 020.7257.3322
Fax - 020.7490.2183
www.colmc.org.uk

Disabled Resources - Canada

Canadian Hard of Hearing Association
2435 Holly Lana
Suite #205
Ottawa, Ontario, Canada
K1V 7P2
voice: 613.526.1584
TTY:613.526.2692
Fax: 613.526.2692
Toll Free: 1.800.263.8068 (In Canada)
E-Mail: chhanational@chha.ca

Canadian Abilities Foundation
340 College Street, Suite #401
Toronto, ON, Canada
M5T 3A9
Tel - 416.923.1885
Fax - 416.923.9829
info@enablelink.org
www.abilities.ca

CNIB National Office
1929 Bayview Avenue
Toronto, ON, Canada
Tel - 1.800.563.2642
Fax - 416.480.7677
info@cnib.ca
www.cnib.ca

How to use the Internet: Finding Reliable Headache Information

By Brent Lucas, BA, Director, Help for Headaches, London, Ontario, Canada

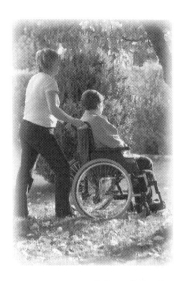

Once we get past the "phobia" of breaking something on our computers, or causing unwanted anxiety, surfing the internet for credible information on headaches can be rewarding and eye-opening. There are many ways to search for information and I will attempt to cover some do's and don'ts.

Like any health information, the internet offers readers a volume of advice, suggestions, and education. I guess that is why it is referred to as the "information super-highway".

First-time users can think of it as going into a large bookstore and scanning the shelves for headache books. Some of you will pick up, scan, and replace a book. Others will read it more thoroughly. Perhaps you will buy a book or newsletter to stay informed on a topic. You may also glance at the book's table of contents or skim the back cover - which often gives you a sense as to what the book is all about and usually a short write-up on the author's credentials, or history. You often have to skim two or three books to get different opinions on a topic.

Using your computer to search for information can be gathered in much the same way. When you use your computer keyboard you can cross-reference articles, keywords, different websites, etc. Using the glossary is as great way to look up terms and compare their meaning as it relates to your field of interest. The glossary and index are located in most books near the back of the book.

On the internet, there are many popular "browsers" that can help you search for a term, topic, city, university, anything. They allow you to do just that - browse. Some examples of internet browsers include www.google.ca, www.yahoo.com, www.hotmail.com, www.alta-vista.com, www.lycos.com . There are many other search engines you can use to find your information that provide similar results. You can locate articles, graphics for your school project, do your banking transactions, email colleagues at work in a different room/building, chat with friends, etc. . from your computer.

At the search menu (most search engines have that option) type in concise keywords, for example: headache groups, headache neurologist's, headache organizations, headache books, headache clinics, etc. If you are pursuing alternative approaches you can use the same method and just search for alternative terms.

Caution: be sure your keywords, doctors, or methods are spelled properly

Try to limit your internet search to 3 or 4 words. If you are in Toronto for example you might try to search for - "headache neurologist's Toronto Canada".
Because so many businesses and health professionals provide information on headaches, one has to be somewhat selective as to the information presented, and as to how credible that information will be. A good rule of thumb is that if the website is linked or endorsed by a headache charity, headache clinic, or the World Headache Alliance, then this is a good indication that the information is credible.

Also headache charities or non-profit groups that are national in scope are very credible. (Canada's national charity is called Headache Network Canada at www.headachenetwork.ca .)

Let's say you typed in www.google.ca and asked the search engine to search for "headache organizations". This is what you would get from the Google search engine.

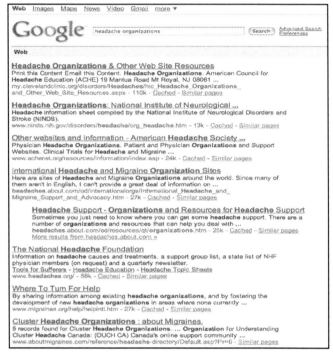

As you can see, you have many options of headache organizations open to you. And almost every webpage that you click and access has links to other credible headache or health websites. The major headache groups, centers, and clinics are found on the Help for Headaches page website at www.headache-help.org and in that page by clicking the "headache links" button from the side menu. Allow yourself a few hours to search for terms as "browsing" can be really a spider-web of information.

Finding trusted sites takes time and research. Like everything else in life, it requires some thought and organization. I caution readers that with a constant "linking system" the sufferer can actually come right back to the place where he/she began. The information is very helpful and can often provide tips on coping strategies, self-help techniques, new and existing medicine suggestions, and alternative treatment approach suggestions.

Most of the time you will receive generic suggestions instead of pointed advice that says - "do this or that". The physician has not seen you nor performed medical tests on you and is therefore limited as to his or her suggestions or advice.

You should not substitute "online advice" for a physician's advice, even though most organizations have researched the problem for years and can generally recommend an expert in the field of headache.

Remember that headaches are classified and diagnosed according to a set of features or symptoms so it is wise for the sufferer to track and record these features as all physician's will ask these important questions. A set of headache questions has been provided for you to fill out and take to your next appointment. See chapter 13 - How to Prepare for your Physician's Appointment.

Remember that the internet, while scary for the beginner can be a wealth of free information to assist you in your quest for finding partial or total relief. Take solace in the fact that there have been many others in similar situations, and there is an established network to aid you in finding solutions. There is still some way to go in terms of treatments but considering the ancient techniques once used, it is safe to say we as a society have come far in our pain control. New headache medicines and techniques are being introduced all the time.

If you cannot afford internet access, here are some tips:

• Almost all libraries now have free internet access for a time limit

• Most headache organizations have internet access through their sign-up systems such as when you donate or subscribe to the membership. They would be more than happy to assist you and may even help research a strategy or term.

• All Universities and Colleges have free internet access and assistance

- Call your public health nurse to see if some local businesses provide free internet access

- Volunteering for charity can give you access to a computer and the internet (that was a hint!)

- Use a friend's system - it is always more fun browsing or exploring these topics with someone to share, and provide feedback. The friend can aid in problem-solving should you get stuck.

If you were to ask someone a question about your headache pattern, expect a generic response as they will not know your neurological history but can point you in the right direction.

Happy clicking!

Editor's Note: Due to page limitations I am not able to publish the many smaller headache organizations, hospitals, centres or clinics. Many of them you will find very useful, as you search. Please refer to www.headache-help.org then click on "Headache Links"

Appendix A

HEADACHE TYPES

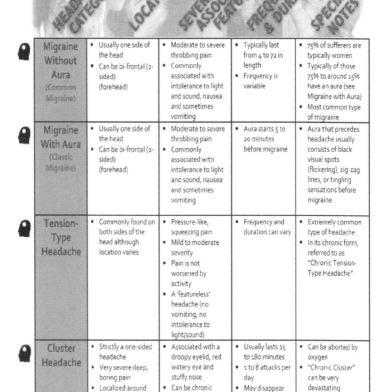

HEADACHE CATEGORIES	LOCATION	SEVERITY & ASSOCIATED FEATURES	FREQUENCY & DURATION	SPECIAL NOTES
Migraine Without Aura (Common Migraine)	• Usually one side of the head • Can be bi-frontal (2-sided) (forehead)	• Moderate to severe throbbing pain • Commonly associated with intolerance to light and sound, nausea and sometimes vomiting	• Typically last from 4 to 72 in length • Frequency is variable	• 75% of sufferers are typically women • Typically of those 75% to around 15% have an aura (see Migraine with Aura) • Most common type of migraine
Migraine With Aura (Classic Migraine)	• Usually one side of the head • Can be bi-frontal (2-sided) (forehead)	• Moderate to severe throbbing pain • Commonly associated with intolerance to light and sound, nausea and sometimes vomiting	• Aura starts 5 to 20 minutes before migraine	• Aura that precedes headache usually consists of black visual spots (flickering), zig-zag lines, or tingling sensations before migraine
Tension-Type Headache	• Commonly found on both sides of the head although location varies	• Pressure-like, squeezing pain • Mild to moderate severity • Pain is not worsened by activity • A 'featureless' headache (no vomiting, no intolerance to light/sound)	• Frequency and duration can vary	• Extremely common type of headache • In its chronic form, referred to as "Chronic Tension-Type Headache"
Cluster Headache	• Strictly a one-sided headache • Very severe deep, boring pain • Localized around the eye	• Associated with a droopy eyelid, red watery eye and stuffy nose • Can be chronic	• Usually lasts 15 to 180 minutes • 1 to 8 attacks per day • May disappear for weeks months at a time	• Can be aborted by oxygen • "Chronic Cluster" can be very devastating • Cluster cycles can last weeks to months

HEADACHE CATEGORIES	LOCATION	SEVERITY & ASSOCIATED FEATURES	FREQUENCY & DURATION	SPECIAL NOTES
Medication Overuse Headache (formerly Rebound Headache)	• Location varies but often experienced on the top of the head	• Mild to moderate in severity of pain • May have migrainous associated features	• Variable but often daily in occurrence • Sometimes 2-3 times per week	• Overuse of Over The Counter (OTC's) or migraine drugs (more than twice a week) are the culprit and other medications are often to blame • Sufferers notice increased medication use with decreased results
Chronic Daily Headache (Mixed Headache)	• Location can vary	• May resemble Tension-Type or Migraine or with features of both	• Often occurs daily • Typically occurs up to 15 days per month	• Medication overuse is often the cause • May be difficult to treat • Often persistent
Sinus Headaches	• Most often facial and cheek area • Blocked nostril	• Acute sharp pain in facial area • Fever is present if true sinusitis • Discharge is usually yellow/green in color	• Quite rare • Frequency is variable	• Depends on treatment type • Rare type of headache • Migraine is often misdiagnosed as Sinus Headache
Headaches in Children	• Often two-sided in younger children • Pain on one side of the head in older children	• Often described as pressure-like • Nausea and vomiting can sometimes bring relief • May have associated features of migraine	• Frequency is variable • Often shorter in duration than those of adults	• Children may complain of fatigue, dizziness • Can be loss of appetite • Recurrent abdominal pain can be a "migraine variant"

Stress
- Stress may trigger a headache, not the cause
- Often let down of a stressful event, causes the headaches

www.headache-help.org

Following done by Dr. Clarence Lay Headache Neurologist New York, NY

World Headache Alliance
www.w-h-a.org

The Headache Institute
New York, NY

Made possible through a contribution by:

MERCK FROSST
Discovering today
for a better tomorrow
www.merckfrosst.ca

This chart is a general guide only - used for educational purposes - please consult a physician with respect to headache

189

Index

A

. . . .

B

. . . .

C

. . . .

D

....

H
....

I
....

K
....

Kern, Ralph, MD. –
   www.headache-help.org/find_a_headache_doctor/ontario.htm

L
....

Lay, Christine, MD –
   www.headache-help.org/find_a_headache_doctor/ontario.htm
lights (fluorescent) pg. 80, 161, 165, 172
lumbar puncture – pg. 99, 149

M
....

magnesium – pg. 59-60, 64-65, 127
Magnetic Resonance Imaging (MRI) - pg. 98-99, 134
MAGNUM – www.migraines.org , pg. 178
massage therapy - pg. 67-68, 78
Mauskop. Alexander, MD – see New York Headache Center
   (Alternative Specialty)
medication overuse headache - formerly Rebound Headache - pg. 116-119
meditation and headache - pg. 82-87
menopause – pg. 131-132, 136-137
menstrual migraine - see migraine/menstrual
Methysergide (Sansert) – no longer available
Michigan Headache & Neurological Institute (MHNI) –
   www.mhni.com , pg. 178
migraine
   -abdominal - see migraine equivalents
   -altitude - see travel
   -auras - pg. 15
   -in children - see children
   -classic (with aura) - pg. 15
   -common (without aura) - pg. 14
   -diary - pg. 171-174
   -equivalents - pg. 18
   -menstrual - pg. 19, 124-131, 172-173
   -non-medication therapies - see non-pharmacological treatments

N
....

O
....

S

....

Saper, Joel, MD – see Michigan Headache & Neurological Institute

secondary headaches - pg. 3, 38-39

self-help strategies - see headache/self-help strategies

serotonin and headache - pg. 7-8, 31, 52

sex-related headache - see coital headache

Shapero, Gary, M.D. –

www.headache-help.org/find_a_headache_doctor.ontario.htm

Sheftell, Fred, M.D. – see New England Center for Headache.

sinus headache - pg. 18-19

sleep disorders - pg. 50, 93, 119, 144, 160, 173

social support - pg. 78-79, 94-96

Solomon, Seymour, MD – see Albert Einstein College of Medicine

South, Valerie, RN – see Headache Network Canada

spinal tap - see lumbar puncture

stress and headache - pg. 37, 144, 160-164

stroke and headache - pg. 23-28, 138-141, 152

Sumatriptan (Imitrex) – pg. 8, 32, 127

support groups - see headache/support groups

symptomatic medicines - see acute medicines

T

....

teeth grinding – pg. 170

temporal arteritis – pg. 152

temporomandibular joint dysfunction (tmj, tmjd) - pg. 22

tension-type headache - pg. 15-16

testing for headache - pg. 97-102

Topiramate (Topamax) – pg. 52-53

travel – pg. 155-160, 165

triggers - see migraine/triggers

triptans - pg. 31-34, 104

tumours – pg. 39

V

....

Valproic Acid (Depakene) – pg. 52-53